（汉英对照）

主编 林 清 胡 颖

中华瑰宝之中医药

Chinese Treasure—
Traditional Chinese Medicine

苏州大学出版社
Soochow University Press

图书在版编目（CIP）数据

中华瑰宝之中医药 = Chinese Treasure—Traditional
Chinese Medicine : 汉英对照 / 林清，胡颖主编 . -- 苏州：
苏州大学出版社 , 2023.9

ISBN 978-7-5672-4400-9

Ⅰ . ①中… Ⅱ . ①林… ②胡… Ⅲ . ①中国医药学—
汉、英 Ⅳ . ① R2

中国国家版本馆 CIP 数据核字（2023）第 165231 号

Zhonghua Guibao Zhi Zhongyiyao
中华瑰宝之中医药
Chinese Treasure—Traditional Chinese Medicine

主　　编：林　清　胡　颖
责任编辑：王　娅

出版发行：苏州大学出版社（Soochow University Press）
地　　址：苏州市十梓街 1 号　邮编：215006
印　　刷：苏州文星印刷有限公司
网　　址：www.sudapress.com
邮购热线：0512-67480030
销售热线：0512-67481020

开　　本：718 mm × 1 000 mm　1/16
印　　张：10
字　　数：154 千字
版　　次：2023 年 9 月第 1 版
印　　次：2023 年 9 月第 1 次印刷
书　　号：ISBN 978-7-5672-4400-9
定　　价：58.00 元

发现印装错误，请与本社联系调换。服务热线：0512-67481020

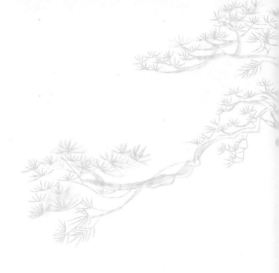

编写人员

主　编：林　清　胡　颖

副主编：贺　芳　顾　垚　盛洁瑾

编　者：（按姓氏笔画排序）

韦姜飞　李梦雯　周　扬

夏　莹　晏锦胜　谈如蓝

主　审：肖　波　顾淑勤

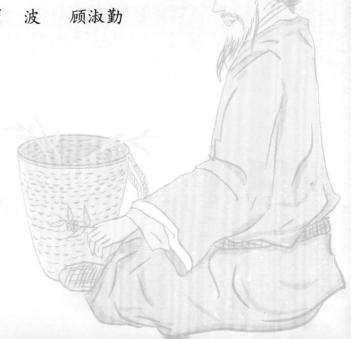

编写说明

2015 年，习近平总书记在致中国中医科学院成立 60 周年贺信中明确指出："中医药学是中国古代科学的瑰宝，也是打开中华文明宝库的钥匙。"传承国粹，弘扬中医药文化，深挖中医药文化的精神内涵和时代价值，充分发挥其作为中华文明宝库钥匙的独特作用，加大中医药文化传播推广力度，推动中医药文化贯穿国民教育、融入群众生活、走向世界舞台是我们出版此书的初衷。

本书用通俗易懂的语言、生动有趣的图片，将深奥难懂的中医药知识理论转变为通俗易懂的科普知识，便于在中小学、社区中宣传和推广。本书采用活页式教材模式，便于使用者根据推广要求选择或组合书本内容，具有灵活多变的可操作性；同时以中英文对照的形式在国际交流中推广中医药文化，提升其海外认可度和接受度。

本书共分为四章。第一章主要介绍中国传统文化、中医药的历史发展以及具有地域特色的"吴门医派"；第二章主要介绍中医基础理论与中医诊疗的过程；第三章主要介绍常见中药材及其在日常生活中的使用等；第四章主要介绍中医适宜技术，如针刺疗法、灸法、传统养生功法等。

本书由林清拟定大纲，组织贺芳、顾垚、韦姜飞、李梦雯、周扬、夏莹、晏锦胜、谈如蓝共同完成中英文内容的编写，再由林清、胡颖、盛洁瑾对中英文进行统稿。本书是多位编者集体智慧的结晶。

苏州卫生职业技术学院肖波副院长、对外合作办公室顾淑勤主任在百忙之中审阅了书稿，并提出宝贵建议，在此表示衷心感谢！

限于水平和能力，书中难免存在疏漏之处，恳请广大读者批评指正。

林清

2023 年 7 月于苏州

目　录

第一章　中国传统文化与中医药

Chapter 1 Traditional Chinese Culture and Traditional Chinese Medicine

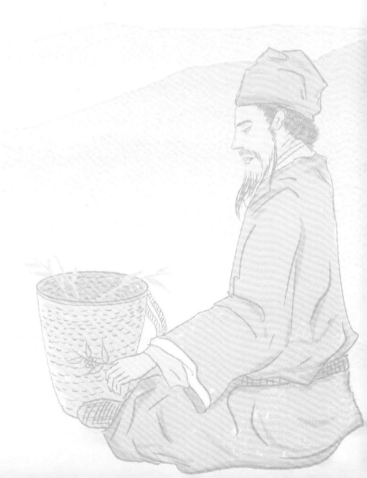

学习情境描述 Learning Situation Description

课堂以讲授为主,配合多媒体教案临床病例(图片资料)示范,并结合相关内容,安排学生分小组相互询问。

Classroom lectures are the main focus, together with the demonstration of clinical cases (pictures) of multimedia teaching plan, combined with relevant contents and arrangements for students to question each other in groups for practice.

学习目标 Learning Objectives

了解中国传统文化、中医药、苏州吴门医派的相关知识。

To learn about traditional Chinese culture, Traditional Chinese Medicine and Suzhou Wumen Medical School.

任务导入 Task Import

一、中国传统文化 Traditional Chinese Culture

中国传统文化是从中华文明演化而成,由居住在中国地域内的中华民族及其祖先所创造的、为中华民族世世代代所继承发展的、具有鲜明民族特色的、历史悠久、内涵博大精深、传统优良的文化。中国传统文化包含哲学思想、琴棋书画、传统文学、传统节日、中国戏曲、中国建筑、中国文字、医药医学、中华武术、饮食厨艺等。

Traditional Chinese culture evolves from Chinese civilization. It is created by the Chinese nation and its ancestors living in China, inherited and developed by the Chinese nation from generation to generation, with distinctive national characteristics, long history, broad and profound connotation and fine tradition. Traditional Chinese culture includes philosophy, *qin*, chess, calligraphy and painting, traditional literature, traditional festivals, Chinese opera, Chinese architecture, Chinese characters, medicine, Chinese martial arts, culinary arts, and more.

儒家、道家
Confucianism, Taoism

1. 哲学思想 Philosophy

中国古典哲学思想主要以儒家思想、道家思想等为代表。

Chinese ancient philosophy is represented by Confucianism, Taoism,etc.

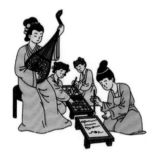

琴棋书画
Qin, chess, calligraphy
and painting

2. 琴棋书画 *Qin*, chess, calligraphy and painting

中国古代的琴棋书画中，"琴"是指古琴、古筝、笛子、二胡等，"棋"是指中国象棋、中国围棋等，"书"是指中国书法，"画"指传统中国画等。

In ancient Chinese *qin*, chess, calligraphy, and painting, "*qin*" refers to ancient *qin*, *guzheng*, flute, *erhu*, etc; "chess" refers to Chinese chess, Chinese Go, etc; "calligraphy" refers to Chinese calligraphy; "painting" refers to traditional Chinese paintings.

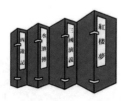

中国四大名著
China's four famous
literary works

3. 传统文学 Traditional literature

中国传统文学多指中国古代的诗、词、曲、小说等多种类型的作品，如《诗经》《西游记》《三国演义》《水浒传》《红楼梦》等。

Traditional Chinese literature refers to ancient Chinese poetry, lyrics, songs, and novels, etc, such as *The Book of Songs, Journey to the West, The Romance of the Three Kingdoms, Outlaws of the Marsh, A Dream of Red Mansions*, etc.

4. 传统节日 Traditional festivals

中国传统节日有春节、元宵节、端午节、中秋节等。

Traditional Chinese festivals include the Spring Festival, the Lantern Festival, the Dragon Boat Festival, and the Mid-Autumn Festival, etc.

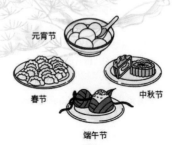

传统节日 Traditional festivals

5. 中国戏曲 Chinese opera

中国戏曲包含京剧、昆曲、黄梅戏等。

Chinese opera includes Peking opera, Kunqu opera, Huangmei opera, etc.

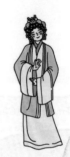

中国戏曲 Chinese opera

6. 中国古代建筑 Ancient Chinese architecture

中国古代建筑具有悠久的历史和光辉的成就。苏州的拙政园、狮子林等是古典园林的代表。

Ancient Chinese architecture has a long history and glorious achievements. Humble Administrator's Garden, Lion Grove Garden, etc. are representatives of ancient Chinese gradens.

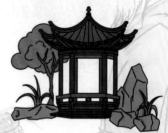

拙政园 Humble Administrator's Garden

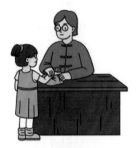

中国文字 Chinese characters

7. 中国文字　Chinese characters

中国有许多种文字，如汉字、藏文、蒙古文字等。

There are many kinds of characters in China, such as Chinese characters, Tibetan characters, and Mongolian characters, etc.

中医 Traditional Chinese Medicine

8. 医药医学　Medicine

在中华五千年的历史长河中，传统医学不仅包含中医，还包含蒙医、藏医等。

In China's 5,000-year-long history, traditional medicines not only include Traditional Chinese Medicine, but also include Mongolian Medicine, Tibetan Medicine, etc.

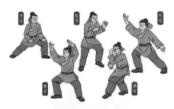

五禽戏 Wuqinxi

9. 中华武术　Chinese martial arts

中华武术是中国古代军事战争传承的一种技术。习武可以强身健体，也可以防御敌人进攻。中华武术包含五禽戏、八段锦、太极拳、少林武术、咏春拳等。

Chinese martial arts is a technique inherited from ancient Chinese military warfare. Practicing martial arts can strengthen the body and also defend against enemy attacks. Chinese martial arts includes Wuqinxi, Baduanjin, Taijiquan, *Shaolin* martial arts, *Yongchun* boxing, etc.

10. 饮食文化　Chinese culinary arts

中华饮食文化素以历史悠远、流传地域广阔、文化底蕴深厚、烹饪工艺卓绝而享誉世界，其中最具代表性的有茶道等。

Chinese food culture is famous around the world for a long history, a wide spread area, profound cultural heritages, and excellent cooking techniques. The famous representatives of Chinese food culture are tea ceremony, wine culture, the Eight Famous Cuisines, etc.

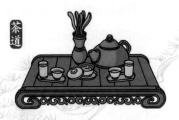

茶道 Tea ceremony

二、中医药 Traditional Chinese Medicine

中医药学是中华优秀传统文化中一颗璀璨的明珠。几千年来，历代医家不断总结中国人民同疾病做斗争的经验和智慧，逐步形成了中医药学深邃的思想、独特的理论和丰富的治法，至今，中医药学仍在中国乃至全世界的卫生保健中发挥着不可替代的作用。

Traditional Chinese Medicine is a bright pearl in China's excellent traditional culture. For thousands of years, doctors of all ages have constantly summarized the experience and wisdom of the Chinese people in fighting against diseases, gradually formed profound ideas, unique theories

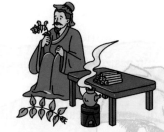

中药 Traditional materia medica

and rich treatment methods of Traditional Chinese Medicine, and made great contributions to the prosperity of the Chinese nation. To this day, Traditional Chinese Medicine still plays an irreplaceable role in health care in China and even the world.

中医特别注重整体观念，不仅认为人体自身是一个有机的整体，体内阴阳平衡、气血和畅、脏腑功能协调就不会生病，就会健康长寿，而且认为人与自然、社会也是一个整体，人们必须顺应四时气候的变化，要"顺四时而适寒暑"，遵循"春夏养阳，秋冬养阴"的养生原则。

Traditional Chinese Medicine pays special attention to the "concept of holism", which believes that the human body itself is a whole organic. If *yin* and *yang* are balanced in the body, *qi* and blood are smooth, and the *zang-fu* organs function in harmony, one will live a long and healthy life. Moreover, man, nature and society are also a whole. People must adapt to the climate change of the four seasons, and follow the health preservation principle of "nourishing *yang* in spring and summer while nourishing *yin* in autumn and winter".

中医重养生，强调"治未病"。何谓"治未病"？"治未病"是指能够早期发现处于萌芽状态的疾病，及时采取各种预防措施，预防病情的发作，包括未病先防和既病防变两个方面。"未病先防"，即防患于未然，摆脱疾病困扰，拥有健康人生。"既病防变"，即如果已经发生疾病，也要积极采取防范措施，防止病情进一步加重。

Traditional Chinese Medicine focuses on health preservation and emphasizes "treating disease before its onset". What is "treating disease before its onset"? It refers to the ability to detect the disease at an early stage and give preventive treatment in time to prevent the onset of the disease. It includes prevention before disease onset and controlling the development of existing disease. "Prevention before disease onset", namely health preservation, means to prevent illness before it occurs, get rid of disease and have a healthy life. "Controlling development of existing disease" means that if a disease has occurred, preventive measures should also be actively taken to prevent further aggravation of the disease.

中药是我国传统药物的总称，是以中医药理论为指导，有着独特的理论体系和应用形式，用于预防和治疗疾病并具有康复与保健作用的天然药物及其加工代用品。中药的应用充分反映了我国历史、文化、自然资源等方面的特点，由于中药的来源以植物类药材居多，使用也最为普遍，所以古时将中药称为"本草"。

Chinese materia medica is the general term of traditional medicine in China. It is a natural medicine, and its processed substitutes are guided by the theory of Chinese medicine, with a unique theoretical system and form of application, used to prevent and treat diseases and have rehabilitation and health care effects. Its application fully reflects the characteristics of China's history, culture, natural resources and other aspects. As its sources are mostly plant-based herbs and their use is the most common, the ancient Chinese medicine was called materia medica.

中医对于疾病的治疗方法极为丰富,除了使用中药外,还有针灸、推拿、功法、拔罐、敷贴、熏蒸等许多有效的非药物疗法。

Traditional Chinese Medicine is very rich in the treatment of diseases. In addition to Chinese materia medica, there are many effective non-drug therapies such as acupuncture, *tuina*, exercise, cupping, application, fumigation.

三、吴门医派 Wumen Medical School

苏州作为我国久负盛名的历史文化名城,建城已 2 500 多年。早在春秋战国时期,苏州就是吴国的都城,以后历为郡、府、省的首府,是江南著名的大都会。这里文化发达,风景优美,温暖湿润,商业繁荣,故有"鱼米之乡"的美誉。丰富的吴文化底蕴给吴中医学的发展增添了活力,也为吴门医派的形成提供了丰厚的文化积淀。

As a famous historical and cultural city in China, Suzhou was built more than 2,500 years ago. As early as the Spring and Autumn Period and the Warring States Period, Suzhou was the capital of the Kingdom of Wu, and later became the capital of counties, prefectures and provinces. It was a famous metropolis in the south of the Yangtze River. With developed culture, beautiful scenery, warmth and humidity, as well as prosperous business, it has the reputation of "land of fish and rice". The rich Wu culture has not only added vitality to the development of Wuzhong medicine, but also provided rich cultural accumulation for the formation of Wumen Medical School.

苏州历朝历代名医辈出，从周朝至今，有记录的名医千余家，其学术成就独树一帜，形成了颇具特色的吴门医派。吴中医家以儒医、御医、世医居多，有较深的文字功底和编撰能力，善于著述、总结前人经验及个人行医心得。

Suzhou has witnessed a large number of famous doctors in the past dynasties. Since the Zhou Dynasty, there are more than 1,000 famous doctors recorded in Suzhou. Their academic achievements are unique, forming a distinctive Wumen Medical School. Most of Wuzhong doctors are Confucian physicians, imperial physicians and physicians from the families for generations. They had a deep knowledge of writing and compiling skills, and were good at writing and summarizing the experience of the predecessors and their personal experience of practising medicine.

苏州是温病学派的发源地，清初叶天士《温热论》的问世更确立了以苏州为中心的温病学派的学术地位。形成了"吴中多名医，吴医多著述，温病学说倡自吴医"的三大特点。这是吴医的精华所在，也是"吴中医学甲天下"的由来。吴门医派为苏州数千年来的繁荣昌盛做出了不可磨灭的贡献。

Suzhou is the birthplace of the school of febrile diseases. The publication of Ye Tianshi's *Treatise on Warm-Heat Diseases* in the early Qing Dynasty established the Suzhou-centred academic status of the school of febrile diseases. This led to the formation of the three main features of the school: "There were many famous doctors in Wu, many works written by Wu doctors, and the doctrine of febrile diseases advocated by Wu doctors." This is the essence of Wu medicine and the origin of "Wu's Chinese medicine is the best in the world". Wumen Medical School has made indelible contributions to the prosperity of Suzhou for thousands of years.

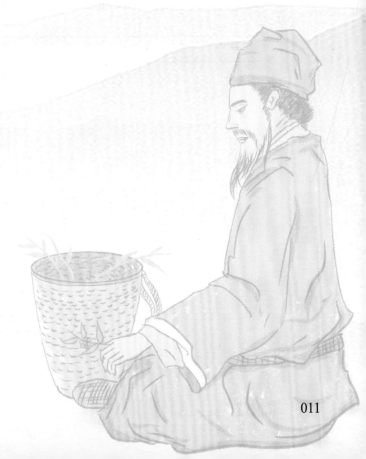

任务分析 Task Analysis

1. 中国传统文化包含哪些内容?

What does traditional Chinese culture contain?

_____

_____

2. 何谓"治未病"?

What is "treating disease before its onset"?

_____

_____

3. 中医非药物疗法有哪些?

What are the non-drug therapies of Traditional Chinese Medicine?

_____

_____

第二章 中国传统医学

Chapter 2 Traditional Chinese Medicine

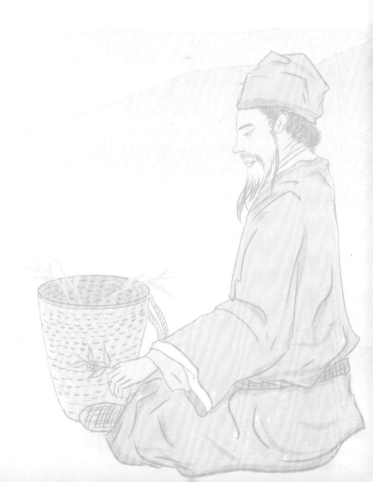

第一节 中医揭示人体的奥秘

Section 1 Traditional Chinese Medicine Reveals Mysteries of Human Body

学习情境描述 Learning Situation Description

课堂以讲授为主，学习并运用中医学基础理论探寻人体的奥秘。

Classroom lectures are the main focus. Learn to apply the basic theories of Traditional Chinese Medicine to explore the mysteries of the human body.

学习目标 Learning Objectives

了解中医学关于五脏、六腑、奇恒之腑的相关知识。

To understand the relevant knowledge of five *zang*-organs, six *fu*-organs and extraordinary *fu*-organs in Traditional Chinese Medicine.

任务导入 Task Import

人体是一个统一而有机的整体，人与自然环境、社会环境都有着密切的联系。中医相信人体的生命活动以五脏为中心，并在此基础上形成了藏象学说。通过各种功能和物质的联系，五脏同六腑、五体、五官、九窍、四肢和躯干形成了一个有机的整体。因此，五脏生理功能之间的平衡协调是维持机体内在环境相对稳定的重要环节。

In Traditional Chinese Medicine, it is believed that the human body is an indivisible organic whole, and it has a close connection with the natural and social environment. It believes that the five *zang*-organs are the core of life activities of the human body. And on this basis, the *Zangxiang* Theory was developed. Through the connection of various functional and materials, the five *zang*-organs form an organic whole with the six *fu*-organs, five body constituents, five scnse organs, nine orifices, four limbs, and the trunk. Therefore, the balance and coordination between the physiological functions of the five *zang*-organs is an important joint to maintain the relative stability of the internal environment of the body.

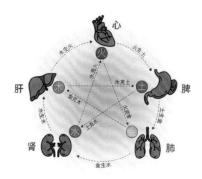

五脏 Five *zang*-organs

值得注意的是，中医学的脏腑与西方实证医学中具象结构的脏器不完全一致，其具有自身的生理和病理理论体系。

It must be pointed out that the names of the viscera of the human body in Traditional Chinese Medicine are not quite similar to those used in modern Western medicine, but many connotations differ between the two systems.

一、何为藏象？ What Is *Zangxiang*?

"藏象"这个词包含了两层意思：

The word "*zangxiang*" contains two meanings.

一是"藏"，即藏于体内的内脏，包含五脏、六腑、奇恒之腑。

One is viscus, which are the viscera hidden in the body, including five *zang*-organs, six *fu*-organs, and the extraordinary *fu*-organs.

臟

五脏 心、肺、脾、 肝、肾	六腑 胆、胃、小肠、 大肠、膀胱、 三焦	奇恒之腑 脑、髓、骨、 脉、胆、女子 胞

五脏，即心、肺、脾、肝、肾。

六腑，即胆、胃、小肠、大肠、膀胱、三焦。

奇恒之腑，即脑、髓、骨、脉、胆、女子胞（子宫、卵巢）。

Five *zang*-organs, namely the heart, the lung, the spleen, the liver, and the kidney. Six *fu*-organs, namely the bile, the stomach, the small intestine, the large intestine, the bladder, and *sanjiao*.

Extraordinary *fu*-organs, namely the brain, the marrow, the bones, the pulse, the bile, the uterus.

二是"象"，指表现于外的生理、病理现象。　**象**

The second is the outward manifestation, which refers to the performance of physiological and pathological phenomena.

五脏的共同特点是化生和储藏精气，六腑的共同特点是受盛和传化水谷，奇恒之腑则两者特点兼有之。

The common characteristic of the five *zang*-organs is to produce and store vital essence, while the common characteristic of the six *fu*-organs is to receive and digest foodstuffs, and transmit and excrete their wastes. The extraordinary *fu*-organs are similar to the *fu*-organs in morphology but store vital essence like and subordinate to the five *zang*-organs.

二、五脏的主要功能 The Main Functions of the Five *Zang*-organs

1. 心 Heart

心脏是五脏中起主宰作用的脏器。它是生命活动的发源地、主神明和血脉的君主之官。

In Traditional Chinese Medicine, the heart is the dominant organ among the five *zang*-organs. It is the cradle of life activities and the charge of mind. It governs the blood like the monarch of the whole body.

（1）心主血脉 Heart's governing the blood

中医学认为血液的正常运行有赖于心脏的正常搏动，这与现代医学对循环系统的认识一致。

That the heart governs the blood means the heart plays a decisive role in the circulatory system by supplying adequate blood to every part of the body. It is similar to the circulatory system in Western modern medicine.

（2）心主神志 Heart's being in charge of the mind

人的精神、意识和思维活动是大脑的生理功能，即大脑对外界事物的反应，但中医学将这部分大脑的功能归属于心脏。

The heart manages all of the mental activities, which includes the mentality consciousness, thinking, emotions, and sensations. The mind actually is the brain's response to external things. But in Traditional Chinese Medicine, this part of the brain's function was ascribed to the heart.

（3）在体合脉，其华在面，开窍于舌 Heart's being in direct communication with the vessels, as reflected in the complexion, and its orifice being the tongue

心功能主要依赖于心气的作用，临床上通过诊察脉象、舌象、面色、胸部感觉等的变化，了解心气的充盈情况。心气充沛的健康人往往面色红润，脉象和缓，舌质淡红。

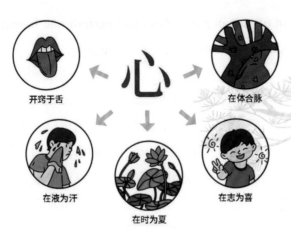

心之联系 Heart connection

It is believed that *qi* of the heart makes the normal heart beat. And the observations of the change of the pulse, the tongue, the complexion and the chest feelings are helpful for us to understand *qi* of the heart. For example, healthy people who are energetic often have ruddy face, mild pulse and light red tongue.

2. 肺 Lung

肺在五脏六腑中所居的位置最高，故有"华盖"之称。

The lung is in the uppermost location of all the *zang*-organs and the *fu*-organs, thus it is called "canopy".

（1）肺主气、司呼吸 Lung's dominating *qi* and controlling respiration

在中医学中，气是构成人体生命物质活动十分重要的精微物质。而肺通过交替地吸入清气、呼出浊气来完成呼吸功能，并调节全身气的升降出入运动，保障人体新陈代谢的正常运行。

In Traditional Chinese Medicine, *qi* refers to the most basic and tiny substances constituting the human body and preserving human life. The lung can regulate the movement of *qi* throughout the whole body to ensure the normal operation of human metabolism and perform the function of breathing by alternately exhaling stale air and inhaling fresh air.

（2）肺主宣发肃降 Lung's dispersing and descending

肺气的一吸一呼带来了宣发和肃降两种气的运动。而这种运动也带来两个方面的改变：一是吸入自然界的清气，排出体内的浊气；二是布散脾所运化的水谷精微至全身，经代谢后，转化为汗液或尿液，排出体外。因此，中医在治疗小便不通的时候常采用宣肺法，这被称为"提壶揭盖"。

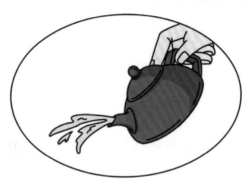

提壶揭盖 "Tihu Jiegai"

Qi of the lung is characterized by dispersing outward and downward. It brings two functions: one is to help the inhalation of fresh air and the elimination of the stale air in the body, the other is to maintain smooth passages for distributing body fluid throughout *zang-fu* organs and tissues under the same dispersing and descending effect. Therefore，we'll treat some of the uroschesis by targeting the lung, so we call this method "Tihu Jiegai".

（3）肺朝百脉，主治节 Lung's toward hundreds of veins, attending section

肺朝百脉并参与宗气的形成，因而肺能助心行血。《黄帝内经》上说："肺者，相傅之官，治节出焉。""相傅之官"即宰相，有辅助君主之意，可见其地位之重要。只有心肺协调，人体的气血循环才能正常，并输送养料维持各脏腑的功能活动。

The lung assists the heart in circulating blood since there are many large blood vessels in the lung, and the lung also participates in the formation of *qi*. The famous book *Huangdi Neijing*（*The Yellow Emperor's Internal Canon of Medicine*）said, "The lung is like a prime minister among the *zang-fu* organs." It means that the lung is very important among the five *zang*-organs. Only when the lung and the heart both function well, can the blood circulation run well, which makes every viscera function well.

（4）在体合皮，其华在毛，在窍为鼻 Lung's being associated with the skin and hair, and having its opening in the nose

肺气功能正常，常表现为皮肤滋润，毛发光泽，鼻窍通利，嗅觉灵敏。而肺气不利时则可出现容易感冒、皮毛枯槁、鼻塞不通、嗅觉减弱等症状。

Traditional Chinese Medicine believes that when *qi* of the lung is functioning well, it is often manifested as moist skin, shiny hair, well-breathing nose and acute sense of smell. When *qi* of the lung is malfunctioning, it can be easy to catch a cold, and have withered skin, blocked nose, weak sense of smell and other symptoms.

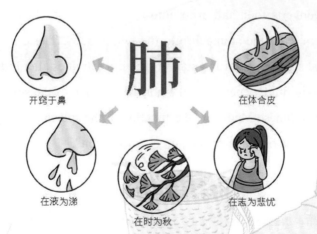

肺之联系 Lung connection

3. 脾　Spleen

中医学中对脾的认识与现代解剖中认定的脾功能差别比较大，其包括了脾脏及胰脏的部分功能，认为脾的主要功能是主运化、升清和统摄血液。

The cognition of the spleen in Traditional Chinese Medicine differs greatly from that in modern anatomy, which includes some functions of the spleen and the pancreas. Its main functions are to govern transportation and transformation, to ascend as well as to control the blood. In Traditional Chinese Medicine, the spleen is the supply station of nutrients.

（1）脾主运化　Spleen's dominating the transformation and transportation

《黄帝内经》中说："脾胃者，仓廪之官，五味出焉。"这说明脾胃是管理粮仓的"官"，负责人体营养的供应。饮食进入胃后，经胃液和胃热的作用，被初步消化，然后需要经过脾的运化功能，将食物中的营养物质及水液布散到全身。人体出生后维持生命活动的基本精微物质，诸如气、血、津液的化生主要依赖于脾的这一功能，所以我们称其为"后天之本"。

Huangdi Neijing said the spleen and the stomach are the "officials" in charge of the granary，which supply the nutrition for the human body. That is, the spleen converts food and drink into refined nutrients. It then absorbs and conveys them from the stomach into the whole body. The production of the essential vital substances for maintaining the life activities after birth, such as *qi*, blood and body fluid, depends on the normal function of the spleen. Therefore, in Traditional Chinese Medicine, the function of the spleen is very important, it is regarded as "the origin of the acquired constitution".

（2）脾主升清　Spleen's ascending function

脾的升清功能使来自食物的气、血、津液上承头面并使部分内脏维持正常位置。如果脾气功能失常则会导致由心、肺、头失养所产生的病理变化，或引起内脏的下垂，表现为心悸、气短、头晕、面色苍白，以及胃、肾、子宫或直肠的下垂。

The spleen's ascending function allows *qi*, blood, and body fluid derived from food and drink to be sent upward to the heart, the lung and the head, and makes some viscera to maintain their correct position. If the spleen is dysfunctional, there may be pathological changes in the body resulting from the lack of nourishment of the heart, the lung and the head, or it may cause ptosis of the internal organs, marked by palpitation, shortness of breath, dizziness, pale complexion, gastroptosis, nephroptosis, prolapse of the uterus or the rectum.

（3）脾主统血 Spleen's controlling blood within the vessels

脾能使血液在脉管内运行，避免血液外溢。

In Traditional Chinese Medicine, we believe the spleen can keep the blood flowing within the vessels, thus preventing blood extravasation.

（4）在体合肌肉，开窍于口，其华在唇 Spleen's dominating the muscles, with its orifice in the mouth, and general condition being manifested in the lips

脾气健运，常表现为肌肉强健有力，口唇红润光泽，食欲正常。

According to Traditional Chinese Medicine, if the spleen functions well, it is often manifested as strong and powerful muscles, rosy lips and normal appetite.

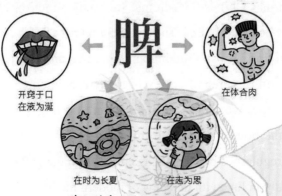

脾之联系 Spleen connection

4. 肝 Liver

肝是贮藏血液的大仓库，主谋虑和藏血的"将军之官"。

The liver is regarded as the great storehouse of blood, like a general who governs the design of strategies.

（1）肝主疏泄 Liver's maintaining the smooth flow of *qi*

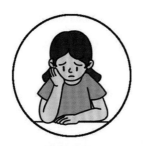 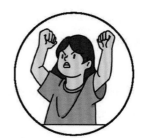

肝气不舒
Discomfort of *qi* of the liver

肝火上亢
Hyperactivity of fire of the liver

肝的主要功能是主疏泄。肝能调畅情志，有主谋虑、藏魄的功能。现代医学认为这些思维意识活动是大脑皮质的功能，但中医将人体出现抑郁或亢奋易怒的病理现象归纳为肝气不舒或肝火上亢的表现，常以调理肝气、平息肝火的方法治疗。肝主疏泄又指肝有疏泄胆汁的功能，可以帮助消化，促进食物的转化，这与现代医学认为肝能分泌胆汁和进行物质代谢的看法基本一致。

In Traditional Chinese Medicine, the main function of the liver is to maintain the smooth flow of *qi*. The liver can adjust the mood, and control the changes of emotion. Those thinking and consciousness activities are thought to be the function of cerebral cortex in modern medicine. But in Traditional Chinese Medicine, we chalk up depression and anger to liver problems. Furthermore, the bile is secreted from the liver in a clear and unobstructed manner and is regularly stored in and excreted from the gallbladder by the liver, which is basically in line with the view of modern medicine.

（2）肝藏血 Liver's storing blood

肝具有贮藏血液的作用，但这种贮藏体现为对全身血量的调节，就如同一个血库一样，现代医学对肝的功能也有同样的认识。

The liver has the function of storing blood, and this storage is reflected in the regulation of blood volume of the whole body. It is just like a blood bank, which seems the same to the liver's function in modern medicine.

（3）在体合筋，其华在爪，开窍于目 Liver's being in charge of the tendons, reflected functionally on the nails, and having its specific orifice in the eyes

肝血充盈，则筋腱有力，运动灵活，能够耐受疲劳。肝与目关系密切，所以肝的功能是否正常，往往可以从眼睛上反映出来。

If the liver is full of blood, then the tendons are strong, and the movement is flexible. The liver can also withstand fatigue. The liver is closely related to the eyes, so whether the liver's function is normal can often be reflected by the eyes.

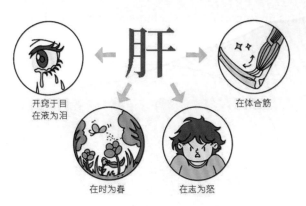

肝之联系 Liver connection

5. 肾 Kidney

《黄帝内经》称肾为"作强之官"。作强，有"精明强干"的意思。中医认为，人体的才智和精巧能力与肾相关。与现代医学中对肾脏的认识局限在泌尿系统不一样的是，中医中的肾包含了生长、发育、生殖及水液代谢部分的内容。

In the book *Huangdi Neijing*, the kidney was called a clever and capable officer. That is because people believe that the intelligence and ingenuity of the human body are associated with the kidney. Unlike the modern medicine, which only makes it an organ of the urinary system, the kidney in Traditional Chinese Medicine is thought to take charge of the reproduction, development, and growth of the body, and the fluid metabolism.

（1）肾藏精 Kidney's storing essence

肾中藏有先天之精，为脏腑阴阳之本、生命之源，所以中医学称其为"先天之本"。中医学认为，机体的生、长、壮、老、死的自然规律，与肾中精气的盛衰密切相关。

There is innate essence hidden in the kidney, which is the source of *yin* and *yang* of the viscera and life. So we call the kidney "the origin of the innate constitution". Traditional Chinese Medicine believes that it is the kidney-essence that plays an important role in human birth, growth, maturity, aging and death.

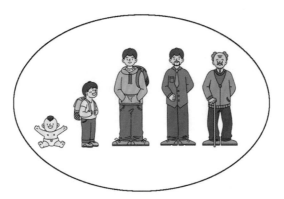

人的生长过程 The process of human growth

（2）肾主水 Kidney's governing water

中医学同样认识到肾与水液代谢的关系，认为肾主水液，提示了肾与尿液生成和排泄的关系。除此以外，作为功能单位的肾与呼吸、神经、内分泌、免疫等系统均有密切关系。

Traditional Chinese Medicine also recognizes the relationship between the kidney and the fluid metabolism, and believes that the kidney governs fluid, suggesting the relationship between the kidney and the production and excretion of urine. In addition, as a functional unit, the kidney is closely related to the respiratory, neurological, endocrine, immune and other systems.

（3）在体合骨生髓，其华在发与齿，开窍于耳及二阴 Kidney's dominating the bone and manufacturing the marrow, being reflected in the teeth and hair, and its body openings in ears, the external genitals and the anus

肾精的强弱可以通过观察骨骼的生长发育、脑的发育、头发的色泽与量、牙齿的坚固情况、耳朵的功能、排泄器官的功能、生殖器官的功能情况来判断。

The strength of the kidney essence can be observed by the bone growth, the brain development, the color and quantity of one's hair, the strength of the teeth, the function of the ears, as well as the function of the excretory organs and the reproductive organs.

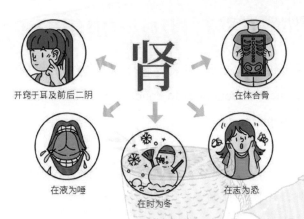

肾之联系 Kidney connection

三、六腑的主要功能 The Main Functions of Six *Fu*-organs

在食物进入人体后，六腑依次履行它们各自的功能。

After the food enters the human body, the six *fu*-organs perform their functions in turn respectively.

胃受纳来自口、咽、食道的食物后，利用它的消磨和腐熟作用，把食物变成食糜。因此，胃被称为"水谷之海"。

The stomach receives food from the mouth, the pharynx and the esophagus, and turns the food into chyme by its grinding and decomposing effect. Therefore, the stomach is called the "reservoir of water and grain".

小肠接下来利用它的分清泌浊的作用，将食糜转化成精微物质和废料。前者由脾转输肺，散布周身；后者中食物残渣下传大肠，水液经三焦下渗至膀胱。

The small intestine then separates the clear from the turbid to convert the chyme into fine matter and waste. The former is transported from the spleen to the lung and distributed throughout the body; the food residue in the latter is transmitted to the large intestine, and the water liquid seeps down to the bladder through the triple energizer.

大肠继续传导食物残渣，并将其转化为粪便经肛门排出。

The large intestine continues to conduct the residue and turn it into feces for excretion through the anus.

胆储藏来自肝脏的胆汁，必要时排泄出胆汁进入小肠和胃，参与食物的消化。此外，中医将胆称为"中正之官"，认为其支配着人体的胆量、决断等精神活动。

The gallbladder stores the bile from the liver, which, when necessary, travels to the small intestine and the stomach to take part in the digestion of food. In addition, Traditional Chinese Medicine refers to the gallbladder as "the official of *zhongzheng*", believing that it controls the human body's mental activities such as courage and decision-making.

膀胱暂时储藏来自肾及三焦的津液，贮存到一定的量，则可随意排出体外形成尿液，履行着"水库主任"的职责。

The bladder temporarily stores body fluid from the kidney and *sanjiao*（triple energizer）, and when it is accumulated to a certain amount, it can be discharged into urine at will, fulfilling the duty of "reservoir director".

三焦则是水液及元气运行的道路。

Sanjiao（Triple energizer）is the pathway through which the water and the primordial *qi* move.

四、奇恒之腑的主要功能 The Main Functions of Extraordinary *Fu*-organs

奇恒之腑形态上类似六腑，却有贮藏生命之精的能力。

The extraordinary *fu*-organs are morphologically similar to the six *fu*-organs, but they have the additional ability to store vital essence.

五、五脏之间的功能联系 The Functional Relationship Between Five *Zang*-organs

中医学认为，正是通过以五脏为中心，并与六腑、奇恒之腑的互相联系所形成的藏象学说，才形成中医学独特的整体观。五脏的生理功能活动不是孤立的，它们通过经络的联系，互相协调，互相配合，共同维持人体正常的生命活动。当这种平衡被打破时，则会形成相应的病理变化。

According to Traditional Chinese Medicine, the unique holistic view is formed by *Zangxiang* Theory, which is centered on the five *zang*-organs and linked with the six *fu*-organs and the extraordinary *fu*-organs. The physiological functions of the five *zang*-organs are not isolated. They coordinate and cooperate with each other through the connection of meridian and collaterals to maintain the normal life activities of the human body. When this balance is broken, the corresponding pathological changes will be formed.

比如，心主血，肺主气，全身血液的循环依靠心气的推动，通过经脉而又聚于肺，经肺的呼吸，进行气体交换，然后再输布到全身，所以只有心肺密切配合，才能使气血运行正常。再比如心与肝，它们都与精神情志活动相关，中医认为，若心肝两脏血虚，则易出现心烦失眠、急躁易怒等精神症状。同理，人体中任何脏与脏、腑与腑、脏与腑之间都存在着不可分割的联系，它们构成了一个统一的整体。

For example, the heart is connected with blood, and the lung is connected with air. Blood circulation needs to be pushed by the heart *qi*, and then blood gathers in the lung, moves through the lung to exchange air, and then distributes throughout the body. Therefore, only good coordination between the heart and the lung can make *qi* and blood run normally. Another example is the heart and the liver, both of which are related to spiritual and emotional activities. Traditional Chinese Medicine believes that if there is blood deficiency in the heart and the liver, anxiety, insomnia, irritability and other mental symptoms will commonly occur. Similarly, in the human body, there is a close connection between the *zang-fu* organs，which forms a unified whole.

任务分析 Task Analysis

1. 请在下列一组图片中选出五脏。

Please pick out the five *zang*-organs in the pictures below.

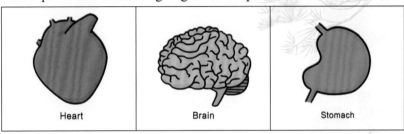

| Heart | Brain | Stomach |

_____ _____ _____

2. 按照藏象学说理论，请将对应脏腑进行分类。

Please classify the corresponding *zang*- or *fu*-organs in the pictures below.

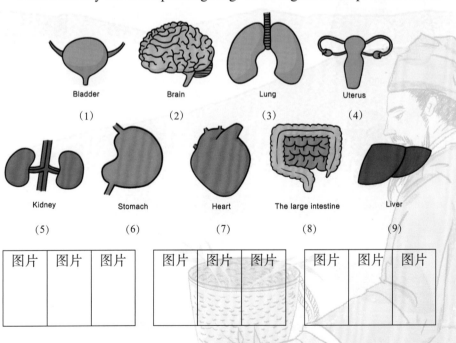

Bladder (1)　　Brain (2)　　Lung (3)　　Uterus (4)

Kidney (5)　　Stomach (6)　　Heart (7)　　The large intestine (8)　　Liver (9)

图片	图片	图片

图片	图片	图片

图片	图片	图片

_____ _____ _____

3. 按照藏象学说理论，将对应部位与五脏连线。

Please match the five *zang*-organs with the corresponding parts.

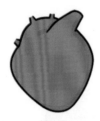

Heart

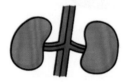

Kidney

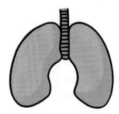

Lung

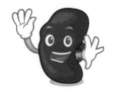

Spleen

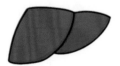

Liver

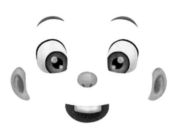

4. 根据藏象学说，结合以下病例病症特点，进行对应连线。

Please match the five *zang*-organs with the corresponding symptoms.

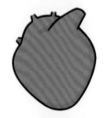

Heart

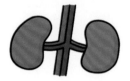

Kidney

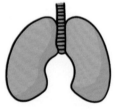

Lung

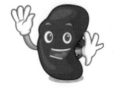

Spleen

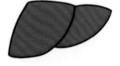

Liver

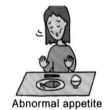

Abnormal appetite

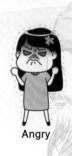

Angry

第二节　中医如何看病

Section 2 The Way Traditional Chinese Medicine Diagnoses Diseases

学习情境描述 Learning Situation Description

课堂以讲授为主，配合多媒体教案临床病例（图片资料）示范，并结合相关内容，安排学生之间进行分组询问实践。

Classroom lectures are the main focus, together with the demonstration of multimedia teaching plan of clinical cases（picture materials）, combined with relevant contents and arrangements for students to question each other in groups for practice.

学习目标 Learning Objectives

掌握与望诊、闻诊、问诊、切诊相关的术语，熟悉四诊的科学表达方式。

To master the common terminologies in inspection, auscultation and olfaction, inquiry, and pulse-taking and palpation, and familiarize with the scientific expression of the four diagnostic methods.

任务导入 Task Import

中医通过望、闻、问、切等诊察方法来审查人体外部征象，分析和明确病因、病性、病位等疾病的本质，从而为辨证论治提供可靠的依据。临床诊病时，医者一定要将四者有机地结合起来，才能客观准确、全面系统地收集病情资料，做出正确的诊断。

Traditional Chinese Medicine examines the external signs of the human body through inspection, auscultation and olfaction, inquiry and palpation (pulse feeling), analyses and clarifies the essence of the disease such as its cause, nature and location, thus providing a reliable basis for diagnosis and treatment. In clinical diagnosis, the practitioner must organically combine the four methods in order to collect information about the disease in an objective, accurate and comprehensive manncr and make a correct diagnosis.

一、望诊 Inspection

望诊是医者运用视觉对患者神、色、形、态等全身情况及局部表现、舌象、分泌物、排泄物等进行有目的的观察，收集病情资料的诊察方法。

Inspection is a diagnostic method to understand the health condition of patients by observing changes in their body's general condition(spirit, color, shape and movement), as well as local manifestations, tongue appearance, secretions, and excretions, and collect disease data.

1. 望神 Inspection of vitality

通过观察人体生命活动的总体表现来诊察病情的方法，其中以望眼神为最重要。临床一般分为"得神""少神""失神""假神"四种。

Inspection of vitality is a method to evaluate the heath conditions by observing the overall manifestations of the human body，particularly the expressions of the eyes. In terms of clinical manifestations, the inspections of vitality can be classified into four patterns: presence of vitality, lack of vitality, loss of vitality and false vitality.

2. 望色 Inspection of complexion

望色指医生通过观察患者全身皮肤（尤其是面部皮肤）的色泽变化来

诊察疾病的方法。面色分为常色和病色。常色指人在正常生理状态下面部的色泽，病色指人体在疾病状态时面部的异常色泽，病色分为青、赤、黄、白、黑五种，分别提示不同脏腑和不同性质的疾病。

Inspection of complexion is a method to diagnose diseases by observing the color changes of the skin, especially the skin of the face, which can be divided into the normal color and the abnormal color. The normal color refers to the color of the human face in its normal physiological state. The abnormal colors are also known as morbid complexion, including changes in both color and luster. Five abnormal colors—bluish, red, yellow, white and black can suggest different disease natures related to different *zang-fu* organs.

以中国人为例，不同的面色与不同的脏腑对应。

Taking the Chinese as an example, different complexion can be observed in the relative *zang-fu* organs.

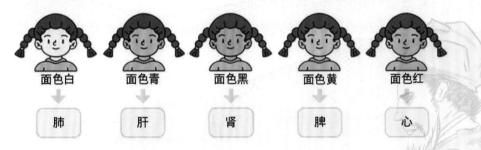

病色与脏腑的对应关系图（面白—肺、面青—肝、面黑—肾、面黄—脾、面赤—心）
The relationship between different complexion and the *zang-fu* organs (white corresponds to the lungs, bluish corresponds to the liver, black corresponds to the kidney, yellow corresponds to the spleen, red corresponds to the heart)

3. 望形体 Inspection of the body building

望形体指通过观察病人的形体及姿态来诊察疾病。望形体主要观察病人形体的强弱、胖瘦等情况。望姿态是指通过观察病人的动静姿态、体位变化及肢体的异常动作来诊察病情。

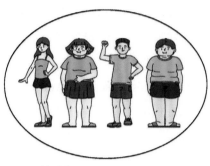

望形体 Inspection of the body

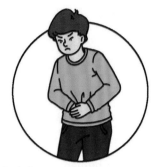

望姿态 Inspection of the posture

This means to observe the patient's body and the posture to diagnose the disease. Inspection of the body mainly observes the strength, weakness, fatness and thinness of the patient's body. Inspection of the posture is to diagnose the disease by observing the patient's dynamic posture, postural changes and abnormal movements of limbs.

4. 望舌 Inspection of the tongue

舌诊，是指通过观察舌质和舌苔的变化，了解机体生理功能和病理变化的诊察方法，是中医望诊的特色之一。

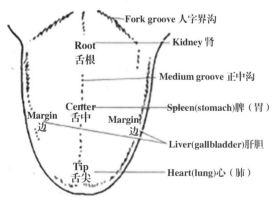

舌诊脏腑部位分属
Correspondence of the tongue to the viscera

Tongue inspection is a method to understand physiology and pathology of the human body by observing the changes of the tongue texture and tongue coating, which is one of the characteristics of inspection in Traditional Chinese Medicine.

望舌质主要包括观察舌体的神、色、形、态和舌下脉络等方面内容。

Inspection of the tongue texture includes the observation of the spirit, color, shape, movement and sublingual veins of the tongue.

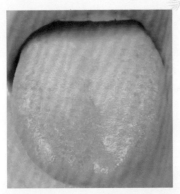

正常舌象 Normal tongue manifestation

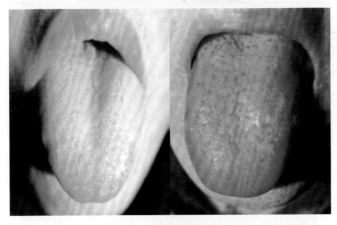

望舌色（淡红舌、红绛舌）
Observing the tongue color (light red tongue, crimson tongue)

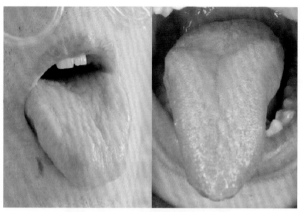

望舌形（胖舌、瘦舌）
Observing the tongue shape (enlarged tongue, thin tongue)

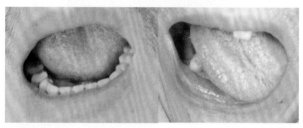

望舌态（痿软舌、歪斜舌）
Observing the tongue movement (flaccid tongue, deviated tongue)

望舌苔主要观察苔质、苔色的变化。

Inspection of the tongue coating mainly observes the changes of the texture and the color of the tongue coating.

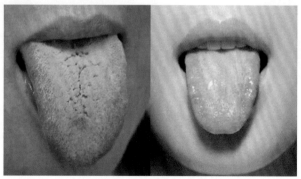

望苔质（厚苔、薄苔）
Observing the texture of the tongue coating (thick coating, thin coating)

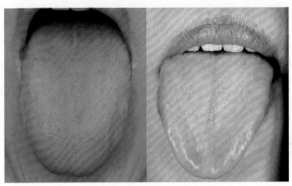

望苔色（白苔、黄苔）
Observing the color of the tongue coating (white coating, yellow coating)

5. 望局部 Inspection of local body parts

根据病情和诊断的需要，对病人的某些部位进行深入、细致的观察，从而帮助了解整体的变化。局部望诊包括望头面、望毛发、望五官、望躯体、望皮肤、望小儿指纹。

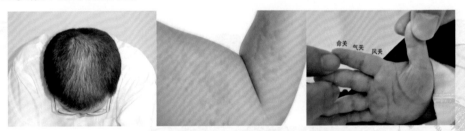

望局部（望毛发、望皮肤、望小儿指纹）
Observing the local body parts (the hair, the skin, the children's finger venules)

According to the needs of the condition and diagnosis, some parts of the patient are observed in depth and carefully to help understand the overall changes. Inspection of local body parts includes looking at the head and the face, the hair, the facial features, the body, the skin, and the children's finger venules.

6. 望排出物 Inspection of excreta

望排出物是通过观察患者的分泌物、排泄物及排出病理产物的形、色、质、量的变化，了解患者各有关脏腑的病变及邪气的性质。

Inspection of excreta means to observe the changes (sputum, thin saliva snivel, thick saliva, etc.) in the shape, color, quality and volume of patients' secretions, discharges and pathological products. This can help with the identification of dysfunctions of the *zang-fu* organs and nature of pathogenic factors as well as disease diagnosis.

二、闻诊 Auscultation and Olfaction

闻诊是医生通过听声音和嗅气味，以诊察疾病的方法。

Through auscultation and olfaction, doctors can diagnose diseases by listening to patients' voice/ sound and smelling the odor of their excreta.

听声音指听患者的声音、呼吸及其他声响。

Auscultation refers to listening to patients' voice, respiration, and other sounds.

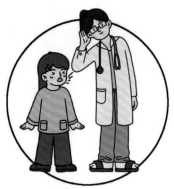

听声音 Listening to patients' sound

嗅气味指嗅病体所发出的各种异常气味及分泌物、排泄物和病室的气味。一般认为声音和气味与人体的生理和病理有关。

Olfaction refers to smelling various abnormal odors emitted by patients' body and the smell of secretions, excreta and their wards. It's believed that changes in voice/sound and odor are related to physiology and pathology of the body.

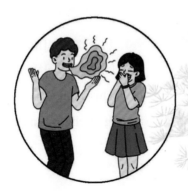

嗅气味 Smelling the odor of patients' excreta

三、问诊 Inquiry

问诊是医生通过对病人或陪诊者进行有目的、有步骤地询问，以了解病情的发生、发展、治疗经过、现在症状和其他与疾病有关的情况，进而诊察疾病的方法。问诊时主要问一般情况、主诉、现病史、既往病史、个人生活史、家族史等。

Inquiry refers to the process to collect information regarding the disease occurrence, progression, previous diagnosis and treatment, and present symptoms by talking to the patients or the persons who accompany the patients. The contents of inquiry include general information, chief complaints, history of present illness, past medical history, personal life history and family history, etc.

问现病史中的现在症状是指对患者就诊时所感到的痛苦和不适以及与其病情相关的全身情况进行详细询问。现在症状是当前病理变化的反映，是诊病、辨证的主要依据。

Inquiry of present symptoms in history of present illness refers to detailed questions of pain, discomfort and related systemic conditions that patients are experiencing during their visit to a doctor. Since present symptoms manifest current pathological changes, they are major clues for disease diagnosis and syndrome differentiation.

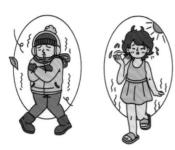

问寒热 Inquiry of chills and fever

1. 问寒热 Inquiry of chills and fever

问寒热指问病人有无怕冷或发热的感觉。

This includes questions regarding patients' feeling of chills and fever.

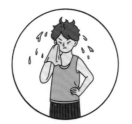

问汗 Inquiry of perspiration

2. 问汗 Inquiry of perspiration

问汗时，应注意了解患者有汗无汗，出汗的时间、部位、多少及其兼症等。

Questions regarding perspiration include the presence, time, location and amount of sweating as well as accompanied symptoms.

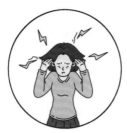

问疼痛 Inquiry of pain

3. 问疼痛 Inquiry of pain

问疼痛，主要询问疼痛的性质、部位、严重程度、时间和伴随症状等。

Inquiry of pain is to ask about the nature, location, severity, time of onset of the pain as well as the accompanied symptoms.

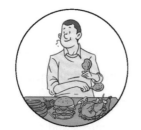

问饮食与口味 Inquiry of food and taste

4. 问饮食与口味 Inquiry of food and taste

问饮食与口味包括问食欲、食量、口渴及口味等。

Inquiry of food and taste includes asking about the appetite, food intake, thirst and taste.

5. 问睡眠 Inquiry of sleep

问睡眠主要询问睡眠时间的长短、入睡的难易、是否易醒、有无多梦等情况，睡眠失常有失眠和嗜睡两种情况。

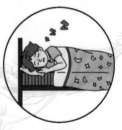

问睡眠
Inquiry of sleep

Asking about sleep mainly asks about the length of sleep time, the difficulty level of falling asleep, whether it is easy to wake up, and whether there are multiple dreams. There are two main sleep disorders: insomnia and somnolence.

6. 问二便 Inquiry of defecation and urination

问二便，应注意询问二便的性状、颜色、气味、时间、便量、便次、排便感觉及兼有症状等。

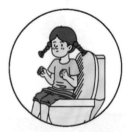

问二便 Inquiry of
defecation and urination

Questions regarding defecation and urination should focus on the property, color, smell, amount, time, frequency, sensation of defecation and accompanied symptoms.

7. 问妇女 Inquiry of gynecology conditions

在问诊女性病人时，除了解一般情况外，尤应注意询问月经、带下、生育情况等，以全面收集病情资料及诊察妇科疾病。

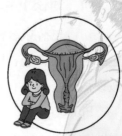

问妇女 Inquiry of
gynecology conditions

When female patients are inquired, in addition to understanding the general situation, special attention should be paid to menstruation, vaginal secretions, and fertility, so as to comprehensively collect disease information and diagnose gynecological diseases.

8. 问男子 Inquiry of andrology conditions

对男子的询问应注意询问其是否有排泄精液等方面的异常情况。

When asking a man, we should pay attention to whether he has abnormal conditions such as excretion of semen.

9. 问小儿 Inquiry of pediatric conditions

询问婴幼儿病情比较困难，主要依靠其亲属提供。除一般问诊外，还须根据小儿的特点，询问出生前后情况、预防接种、传染病史，以及是否受到惊吓等。

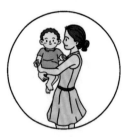

问小儿 Inquiry of pediatric conditions

It is difficult for infants and children to be inquired about their conditions. Information can be got mainly from their parents. In addition to the general consultation, according to the characteristics of them, it is also necessary to ask about the situation before and after their birth, the vaccination, the history of infectious diseases, and whether they are frightened.

四、切诊 Pulse Taking and Palpation

切诊包括脉诊和按诊两个部分，是医生用手在病人身体的一定部位上进行触、摸、按、压，以诊察病情的方法。其中脉诊是切按患者的脉搏，按诊是对患者的手足、肌肤、胸腹、腧穴等有关部位的按压。

Pulse taking and palpation includes two parts: pulse diagnosis and palpation diagnosis. It is a method in which the physicians touch, feel, push and press certain parts of the patient's body with their hands to observe the condition of the patient. Pulse-diagnosis is the pressing of the patient's pulse; palpation diagnosis is the pressing of the patient's hands and feet, skin, chest and abdomen, acupuncture points and other relevant areas.

1. 脉诊 Pulse diagnosis

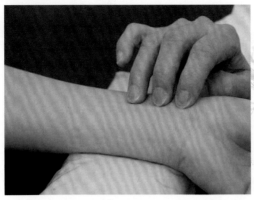

寸口诊法 Diagnosis in Cunkou area (radial artery)

脉诊是医生以指腹切按患者动脉搏动，以探测脉象、了解病情的诊断方法。脉诊历来有多种，现在常用的是"寸口诊法"，即切按病人腕后桡动脉搏动明显处。平脉指正常人在生理条件下出现的脉象。脉象的辨别常通过位、数、形、势四个方面来进行，脉象根据不同的特点基本分类有 28 种。

Pulse diagnosis is a method to examine medical conditions and identify syndromes by feeling the patient's pulse with the fingers. There have always been many kinds of pulse diagnosis. The commonly used method is the "Diagnosis in Cunkou area（radial artery）", because the incision of the patient's posterior wrist radial artery is obviously pulsating. Physiologically, a normal pulse is seen in healthy people. Generally, pulses are identified by four aspects, which are location, frequency, shape and strength. There are altogether 28 basic classifications according to the different characteristics of the pulse.

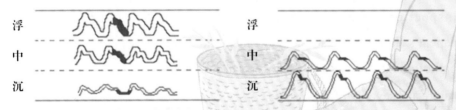

浮脉与沉脉 Floating pulse and deep pulse (location)

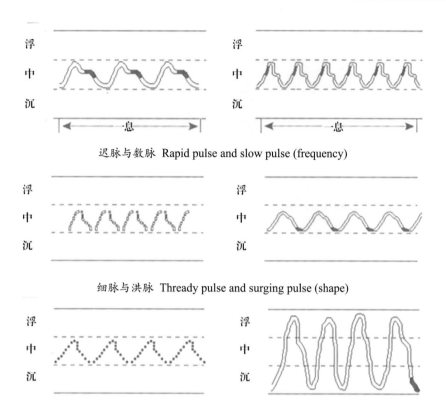

迟脉与数脉 Rapid pulse and slow pulse (frequency)

细脉与洪脉 Thready pulse and surging pulse (shape)

虚脉与实脉 Deficient pulse and excess pulse (strength)

2. 按诊 Body palpation

按诊是对病人的肌肤、手足、脘腹及其他病变部位施行触摸按压，从而推断疾病病位、性质和疾病轻重等情况的一种诊察方法。

Palpation diagnosis is a diagnosis and inspection method to touch and press the patient's skin, hands and feet, abdomen and other pathological parts, so as to infer the location, nature and severity of the disease.

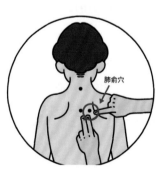

按腧穴 Palpation of acupuncture points

任务分析 Task Analysis

1. 医生可以主要通过哪几种途径了解患者？

What are the main ways to understand the patient when he/she comes to the doctor ?

_____

_____

2. 医生要观察患者哪些方面（望诊）？

What aspects of the patient will be observed (inspection) by doctors ?

_____

_____

3. 医生通常可以从哪几个方面询问患者情况（问诊）？

Which aspects should the doctor ask about the patient (inquiry) ?

_____

_____

4. 切诊分为哪两个部分？

What are the two parts of palpation?

_____

_____

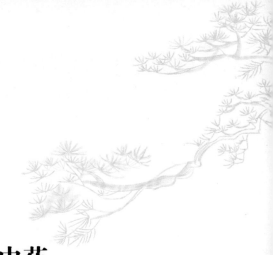

第三章 中药

Chapter 3 Chinese Materia Medica

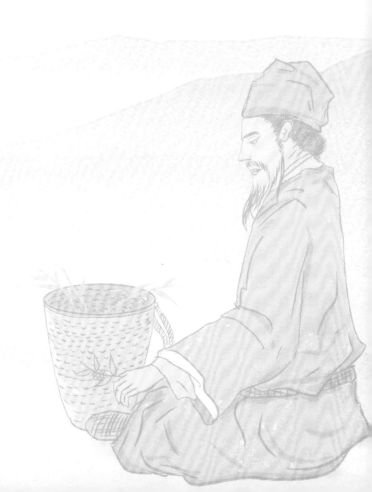

第一节 认识中药材

Section 1 Learning about Chinese Medicinal Materials

参观中药科普馆，认识常见的中药材。

Visit the Museum of Chinese Materia Medica and learn about common Chinese medicinal materials.

掌握中药的概念，了解常见中药材和中成药，能认识一些常见中药材。

To grasp the concept of Chinese materia medica, to understand common Chinese medicinal materials and Chinese patent medicine, as well as to know some common Chinese medicinal materials.

两千多年来，中医药为中华儿女的繁衍昌盛发挥了巨大作用。新冠疫情曾在全球肆虐，中药被广泛使用在抗疫的各个阶段。中药是我国传统药物的总称，是在中医药理论指导下认识和使用的药物。由于中药材的来源以植物类药材居多，使用也最为普遍，所以古时将中药称为"本草"。"本草"为"本之自然"的意思。《说文解字》中对"药"的解释是"治病草"，即为苦痛的病人解困救治，只因草木有情、虫石有性。

For more than 2,000 years, Traditional Chinese Medicine has played a huge role in the reproduction and prosperity of Chinese people. When the COVID-19 pandemic was raging around the world, Chinese materia medica is on the front line of fighting against the pandemic. Chinese materia medica is a general term for our traditional medicine, which is recognized and used under the guidance of the theory of Traditional Chinese Medicine. Since Chinese medicinal materials are mostly derived from plant-based herbs, they were known in ancient times as materia medica. Materia medica (*bencao*) means "original nature". In the book *Shuo Wen Jie Zi*, the word "medicine" is interpreted as a "healing herb", which is used to relieve the suffering patients, simply because grasses and trees have feelings and insects and stones have nature.

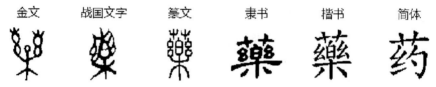

| 金文 | 战国文字 | 篆文 | 隶书 | 楷书 | 简体 |

"药"的字形演变 Glyph evolution of the character 药

在原始社会，人类就有了简单的医疗活动。人们在寻觅食物时常常会因误食而发生致病或中毒，有时也会因为偶然吃了一些"食物"，使原有病症减轻,甚至消除。在长期的经验积累下,人们逐渐发现并开始使用药物,因此也有了"药食同源"的说法。现代常用中药中仍然有一些药物既可以作为中药，也可以作为食材，如薏苡仁、芡实、枸杞子等。

In primitive society, human beings had simple medical activities. When people searched for food, they would often get sick or poisoned by mistake, or sometimes they would eat some "food materials" by chance, which would alleviate or even eliminate their existing illnesses. With the accumulation of experience over time, people gradually discovered and began to use medicines, hence there is also the saying that "food and medicine share the same source". There are still some medicines in common use in modern Chinese materia medica that can be used as both herbs and food ingredients, for example, semen coicis, gordon euryale seed and matrimony vine.

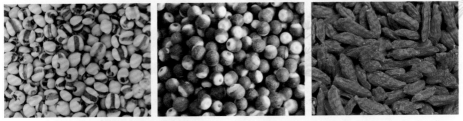

薏苡仁、芡实、枸杞子 semen coicis, gordon euryale seed, matrimony vine

一、道地药材 Genuine Regional Medicinal Materials

道地药材又称"地道药材"，是来自传统产区的质量好、疗效高的中药材。这些药材历史悠久、产地适宜、品种优良、产量丰富、炮制考究、疗效显著，带有地域特点。著名的道地药材包括：四川的黄连、川芎、附子，浙江的白芷、菊花，河南的地黄、牛膝、山药，东北的人参、细辛，山东的阿胶，宁夏的枸杞子，甘肃的当归，等等。

Genuine regional medicinal materials are Chinese medicinal materials of good quality and high curative effect from traditional producing areas. These medicinal materials have a long history, suitable producing area, excellent varieties, abundant yield, exquisite processing, outstanding curative effect, with regional characteristics. For example, Coptis chinensis, Szechwan lovage rhizome and monkshood in Sichuan, radix angelicae, chrysanthemum in Zhejiang, radices rehmanniae, radix achyranthis bidentatae and Chinese yam in Henan, ginseng and asarum in Northeast China, colla corii asini in Shandong, matrimony vine in Ningxia and Chinese angelica in Gansu are all famous genuine regional medicinals.

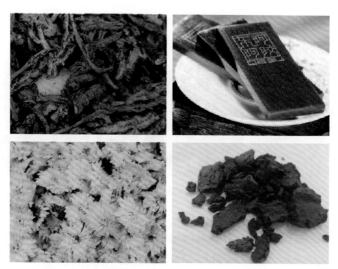

黄连、阿胶、菊花、地黄
Coptis chinensis, colla corii asini, chrysanthemum, radices rehmanniae

二、中药材的采收和炮制　Harvesting and Processing of Chinese Medicinal Materials

中药材的采收季节、时间、方法和贮藏对其品质的好坏有着密切的影响，是保证药物质量的重要环节。因此，药物采收要根据不同的药用部分，有计划地进行采集和贮藏，这样才能得到较高的产量和品质较好的药物，以保证药物的供应和疗效。

The harvesting season, time, method and storage of Chinese herbs are closely related to the quality of Chinese medicinal materials, which is an important factor to ensure the quality of medicine. Therefore, the collection and storage of herbs should be carried out in a planned way according to different medicinal parts, so as to obtain higher yield and medicinal materials of better quality to ensure the supply and efficacy of them.

炮制又称"炮炙""修事""修治"等，是中药特有的加工处理过程，其主要目的是使药物便于制剂和贮存、保证安全用药、增强药物的功能、提高临床疗效、便于服用。炮制中药材的方法有修治、水制、火制、水火共制等。

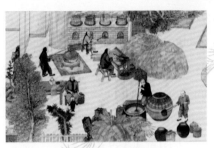

传统中药炮制场景
The processing scene of
Chinese materia medica

Paozhi (medicinal processing, also known as *paozhi*, *xiushi*, and *xiuzhi*, etc.), is a process unique to Chinese materia medica. The main purpose is to facilitate preparation and storage, to ensure safe use of medicines, to enhance the functions of medicines, to improve clinical efficacy and to facilitate administration. The processing methods of Chinese materia medica include processes with water, fire, or water and fire together.

三、常见中药材举例 Examples of Common Chinese Medicinal Materials

1. 人参 Ginseng

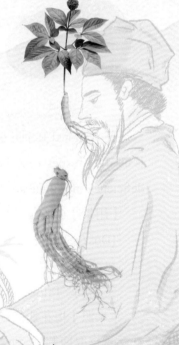

【来源】多于秋季采挖，洗净后晒干或烘干。栽培的俗称"园参"。播种在山林野生状态下自然生长的称"林下山参"。

[Source] Often excavated in autumn, drying in the sun or oven after washed. The cultivated ones are commonly known as "garden ginseng"; the ones sowing in the wild state of the mountain and growing naturally are called "forest ginseng ".

【主要功用】人参具有补气，复脉，补脾补肺，养血，安神的作用，可以用于治疗虚脱，脉搏微弱，食欲缺乏，肺虚咳喘，口渴，发热，气血亏虚，久病虚弱，心悸，失眠等。

[Functions] Ginseng is used to tonify the

人参 Ginseng

original *qi*, resume pulse, tonify the spleen and the lung, nourish blood, and tranquilize the mind. It is used for body deficiency, faint pulse, low appetite, dyspnea and cough caused by lung deficiency, thirsty caused by fluid damage, interior heat, deficiency of *qi* and blood, frail caused by long term illness, fright palpitations, and insomnia, etc.

【用量】3~9 g。

[Dosage] 3~9 g.

2. 灵芝 Reishi

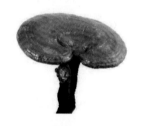

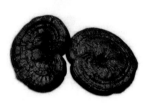

灵芝 Reishi

【来源】全年采收的环境中，除去杂质，剪除附有朽木、泥沙或培养基质的下端菌柄，阴干或在 40℃ ~50℃的环境中烘干。

[Source] Harvest throughout the year. Remove impurities, cut off the fungus stalks attached with rotten wood, silt or substrate, and dry in the shade or at 40℃–50℃.

【主要功用】灵芝是一味补气药物，可以镇静神经，缓解咳嗽和哮喘。常用于治疗烦躁不安、失眠心悸、肺虚、咳嗽哮喘、虚乏气短、食欲缺乏等。

[Functions] Reishi can tonify *qi*, calm nerves, relieve cough and asthma. It is used for restlessness, insomnia, palpitation, lung deficiency, cough and asthma, deficiency of fatigue and shortness of breath, and the lack of appetite, etc.

【用量】6~12 g。

[Dosage] 6~12 g.

3. 鹿茸 Pilose antler

【来源】梅花鹿的幼角习称"花鹿茸"，马鹿的幼角习称"马鹿茸"。夏、秋两季锯取鹿茸，经加工后，阴干或烘干。

[Source] The young antler of sika deer without ossification is known as " sika deer's pilose antler ", while the young antler of red deer without ossification is known as " red deer's pilose antler". In summer and autumn, pilose antler is sawed and dried in the shade or oven.

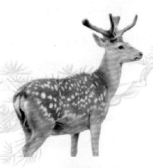

【主要作用】鹿茸具有健肾阳，养精血，强筋骨，调理冲任，托疮毒的作用，可以用于治疗肾阳不足、血虚、阳痿、宫冷不孕、消瘦、乏力、畏寒、眩晕、耳鸣、耳聋、腰脊冷痛、筋骨痿软、月经不调、坏疽不敛等症状。

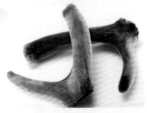

鹿茸　Pilose antler

[Functions] Pilose antler can strengthen kidney *yang*, nourish blood, strengthen muscles and bones, regulate *chongren*, stop sore poison. It is used for deficiency of kidney *yang*, deficiency of blood, impotence and asthenia, uterine cold, infertility, emaciation, fatigue, fear of cold, vertigo, tinnitus, deafness, cold pain of waist and spine, muscle and bone impotence, irregular menstruation, etc.

【用量】1~2 g。

[Dosage] 1~2 g.

4. 薄荷 Mint

【来源】夏、秋二季茎叶茂盛或花开至三轮时，选晴天，分次采割地上部分，晒干或阴干。

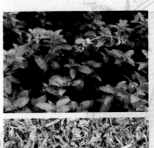

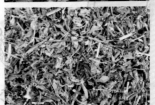

[Source] In summer and autumn, when the stems and leaves are flourishing or flowers bloom to three rounds, pick and cut them in sunny days in different times, and then dry in the sun or dry in the shade.

薄荷　Mint

【主要作用】薄荷具有疏散风热，清利头目，利咽，透疹，疏肝行气的作用，可以用于治疗风热感冒、风温初起、头痛、眼睛红肿、咽喉肿痛、口疮、风疹、麻疹、胸胁胀痛。

[Functions] Mint can evacuate wind heat, clear the mind, benefit pharynx, penetrate rash, and soothe the liver and *qi*. It is usually used for wind-heat cold, wind-temperature onset, headache, eye red, throat obstruction, mouth sore, rubella, measles, chest and hypochasm distension.

【用量】3~6 g。

[Dosage] 3~6 g.

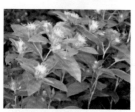

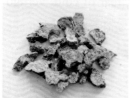

苍术 Rhizoma
atractylodis

5. 苍术 Rhizoma atractylodis

【来源】春、秋二季采挖，除去泥沙，晒干，撞去须根。

[Source] In the spring and autumn, dig it, remove the sediment, and then dry and knock out the roots.

【主要功用】苍术是一味常用的化湿药，可以用于治疗多种类型的腹泻、皮肤瘙痒等，也可以用来预防感冒。

[Functions] Rhizoma atractylodis is a commonly used medicine for resolving dampness. It can be used to treat many types of diarrhea, itchy skin, etc., and can also prevent colds.

【用量】3~9 g。

[Dosage] 3~9 g.

四、中成药简介 Introduction to Chinese Patent Medicine

中成药是指经药品监督管理部门批准、在中医药理论指导下生产和应用、可以直接在市场上销售的具有一定质量规格的中药制剂成品。中成药一般应具有特定的名称和适当的包装，在标签和说明书上标有批准文号、品名、规格、成分、含量、功能主治、临床应用、用法用量、禁忌与注意事项、生产批号等。在中成药中，非处方药是患者不需要医生的处方就可以直接购买并使用的。

Chinese patent medicine refers to the finished Chinese medicine preparations with certain quality of them are approved by the drug regulatory department and produced and applied under the guidance of the theory of Traditional Chinese Medicine. As a special commodity entering the circulation field, Chinese patent medicine should generally have a specific name, appropriate packaging, and be marked with approval number, product name, specifications, ingredients, content, functions, clinical application, usage and dosage, contraindications and precautions, production batch number, etc. on the label and instructions. Among them, over-the-counter Chinese patent medicine can be directly purchased and used by patients without doctor's prescription.

1. 六味地黄丸 Liuwei radices rehmanniae pill

【主要功用】六味地黄丸是补肾阴的常用药，可以用于治疗慢性肾炎、高血压、糖尿病、肺结核、更年期综合征等疾病中的头晕目眩、腰膝酸软、口渴等症状。

[Functions] Liuwei radices rehmanniae pill is a commonly used medicine to tonify kidney *yin*. It can be used to treat chronic nephritis, hypertension, diabetes, tuberculosis, menopausal syndrome and other diseases in which there are symptoms such as dizziness, waist and knee weakness, and thirst.

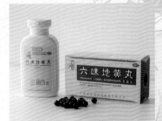

六味地黄丸 Liuwei radices rehmanniae pill

2. 川贝枇杷膏 Chuanbei loquat paste

【主要功用】川贝枇杷膏是止咳化痰的常用药，可以用于治疗因支气管扩张、肺脓疡、肺心病、肺结核等疾病而导致的咳嗽有黄痰、咽喉肿痛

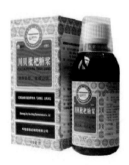

川贝枇杷膏 Chuanbei loquat paste

等症状。

[Functions] Chuanbei loquat paste is a commonly used medicine for relieving cough and resolving phlegm. It can be used to treat symptoms such as cough with yellow sputum and sore throat in bronchial dilatation, lung abscess, pulmonary heart disease and tuberculosis.

任务分析 Task Analysis

1. 请在图片下方写出图片中药材的中英文名称。

Write down the Chinese and English name of the Chinese medicinal materials in the following pictures.

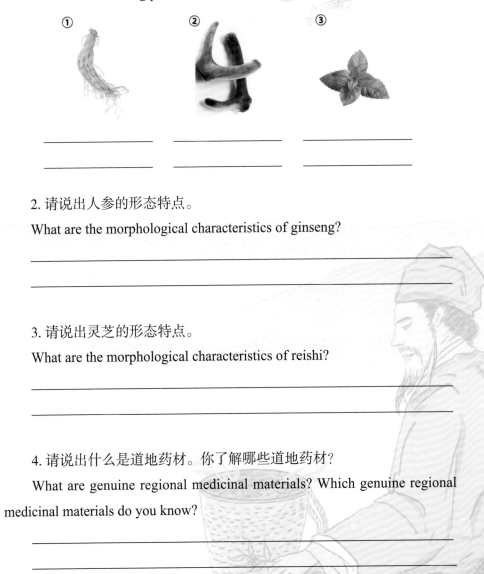

①   ②   ③

_____ _____ _____

_____

2. 请说出人参的形态特点。

What are the morphological characteristics of ginseng?

_____

_____

3. 请说出灵芝的形态特点。

What are the morphological characteristics of reishi?

_____

_____

4. 请说出什么是道地药材。你了解哪些道地药材？

What are genuine regional medicinal materials? Which genuine regional medicinal materials do you know?

_____

_____

第二节　药补不如食补

Section 2　Tonic Food Is Better than Tonic Medicine

学习情境描述 **Learning Situation Description**

根据药膳制作方法，在中药炮制实训室制作时令药膳。

Prepare seasonal medicinal diet in the processing training room of Chinese materia medica according to the preparation method of medicinal diet.

学习目标 **Learning Objectives**

了解药膳的常见基础理论，会制作一道时令药膳。

To understand the common basic theories of medicinal diet, and to be able to make a seasonal medicinal diet.

任务导入 **Task Import**

在我国博大精深的中医药文化体系中，药食同源的概念形成已久，即药物和食物均来源于自然界。早在为了生存而摄取食物的远古时代，人类就发现一些食物在果腹的同时还具有增强体质、减少或缓解疾病的作用。这使人类从偶然发现转变为主动寻求，这种寻求的本能和经验的积累在之后的生活实践中逐步形成了药膳的雏形。

In China's extensive and profound Traditional Chinese Medicine cultural system, the concept of medicine and food sharing the same origin has been

065

formed for a long time, that is, medicine and food are both derived from nature. As early as in the era of food intake for survival, human beings have found that some foods, while filling their stomachs, also have the effect of strengthening physical fitness, and reducing or even alleviating diseases. This makes accidental discovery turn into active seeking. This seeking instinct and accumulation of experience gradually formed the rudiment of medicinal diet in the future life practice.

一、中药药膳 Chinese Medicinal Diet

中药药膳，指在中医药理论指导下，将适宜的中药材与食物进行合理的配伍，采用传统制作工艺和现代科学加工制作技术，烹饪制作成既能果腹，满足人们对美食的追求，又具有保健、预防、治疗作用，可用于防病治病、强身益寿的特殊膳食品。

Chinese medicinal diet refers to the reasonable compatibility of suitable Chinese medicinal materials and food. Under the guidance of Traditional Chinese Medicine Theory, with traditional production technology and modern scientific processing and production technology, it is cooked and made into a special diet that can not only satisfy people's pursuit of delicious food, but also have the functions of health care, prevention and treatment, which can be used for disease prevention and treatment, physical fitness and longevity.

二、常见药膳原料 Common Ingredients of Chinese Medicinal Diet

（一）中药类原料 Raw materials of Chinese medicinal

药膳除了需要具有一定的养生作用和食疗作用外，还应考虑实用性和安全性，因此并非所有的中药材都可以用于烹制药膳。严格地讲，可用于药膳的中药必须达到以下要求：口感与口味适合于烹饪，易被人们接受；对药膳风味影响不大，或通过烹饪加工能达到一定风味要求；安全有效。山药、山楂、甘草、肉桂、百合等都是常见的药膳原料。

Medicinal diet, in addition to the need to have a certain health and therapeutic effect, should also consider practicality and safety. Therefore, not all Chinese medicinal materials can be used to cook medicinal diet. Strictly speaking, Chinese medicinal materials that can be used in medicinal diet refer to those that are suitable for cooking, easily accepted by people, or have little impact on the flavor of medicinal diet, or can meet certain flavor requirements through cooking and processing, and at the same time, safe and effective. For example, Chinese yam, fructus crataegi, licorice root, cinnamon, Lilium brownii and so on.

1. 肉桂　Cinnamon

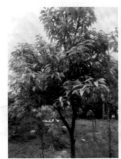 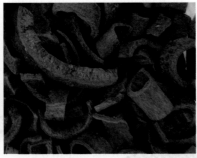

肉桂　Cinnamon

【来源】肉桂为樟科植物肉桂树的干燥树皮，多于秋季剥取，阴干。

[Source] This product is the dried bark of the cinnamomum cassia, mostly peeled in autumn and dried in the shade.

【主要功用】肉桂是一味常用的温里药，可以用于治疗支气管哮喘、慢性支气管炎、腰痛、荨麻疹等。

[Functions] Cinnamon is a commonly used interior-warming medicinal material. It can be used to treat bronchial asthma, chronic bronchitis, low back pain, urticaria, etc.

【用量】1~5 g。

[Dosage] 1~5 g.

2. 山楂 Fructus crataegi

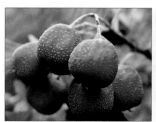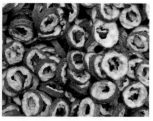

山楂 Fructus crataegi

【来源】山楂为蔷薇科植物山里红或山楂树的成熟果实。秋季果实成熟时采收、切片、干燥。

[Source] This product is the ripe fruit of Crataegus pinnatifida Bge. var. major N.E.Br. or hawthorn Crataegus pinnatifida Bge. of the Rosaceae plant. They are harvested in autumn when the fruit is ripe, and then sliced and dried.

【主要功用】山楂是一味常用的消食药。常用于治疗消化不良、冠心病、心绞痛、高脂血症、动脉粥样硬化等。

[Functions] Fructus crataegi is a commonly used digestant medicinal material. It can often be used to treat dyspepsia, coronary heart disease, angina, hyperlipidemia, atherosclerosis and so on.

【用量】9~12 g。

[Dosage] 9~12 g.

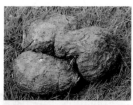
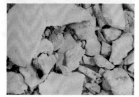

茯苓 Poria cocos

3. 茯苓 Poria cocos

【来源】茯苓为多孔菌科真菌茯苓的干燥菌核。多于7月到9月间采挖，挖出后除去泥沙，堆置"发汗"，反复数次至现皱纹、内部水分大部分散失后阴干，称为"茯苓个"；或将鲜茯苓按不同部位切制，阴干，分别制成"茯苓皮"及"茯苓块"。

[Source] This product is a dried sclerotium of Poria cocos, a fungus of the family polyporaceae mostly dug from July to September, removing sediment after digging, and stacking for "sweating". This process is repeated several times until the wrinkles appear, and most of the internal moisture loss, and then they are dried in the shade, called "Poria cocos"; or the fresh Poria is cut and dried in the shade according to different parts, called "Poria cocos skin" and "Poria cocos block" respectively.

【主要功用】茯苓是一味常用的利水药。可以用于治疗多种水肿、幼儿腹泻等。

[Functions] Poria cocos is a commonly used diuretic medicine. It can be used to treat a variety of edema, infantile diarrhea, etc.

【用量】10~15g。

[Dosage] 10~15g.

4. 芡实 Gordon euryale seed

【来源】本品为睡莲科植物芡的干燥成熟种仁。秋末冬初采收成熟果实，除去果皮，取出种子，洗净，再除去硬壳（外种皮），晒干后制成。

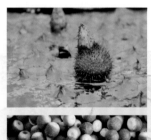
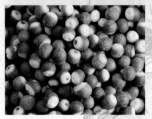

[Source] This product is the dried mature seed kernels of Euryale ferox Salisb in Nymphaeaceae family. Ripe fruits are harvested in late autumn and early winter. Remove the peel, take out the seeds, wash them, and then remove the hard shell (outer seed husk) and dry in the sun.

芡实 Gordon euryale seed

【主要作用】芡实是一味收涩药，可以补肾、补脾，常用于治疗遗精、遗尿、腹泻等。

[Functions] Gordon euryale seed is an astringent medicine. It can tonify the kidney and the spleen, and it is used to treat spermatorrhea, enuresis, diarrhea, etc.

【用量】9~15g。

[Dosage] 9~15g.

（二）食物类原料 Food ingredients

中医药学自古以来就有"药食同源"的说法。《黄帝内经太素》说："空腹食之为食物，患者食之为药物。"许多食材既是食物，也是药物，食物和药物一样能够用来防治疾病。食物类原料一般包括粮食类、蔬菜类、野菜类、食用菌类、果品类、禽肉类、畜肉类、蛋奶类、水产类、调味品、佐料等。以下简要介绍一些常见食物类原料。

Since ancient times, there has been a saying in Traditional Chinese Medicine that "medicine and food share the same origin". It is stated in *Huangdi Neijing-Tai Su* that ordinary food is food, and patients' food is medicine. Many ingredients are both food and medicine, and food, like medicine, can be used to prevent and treat diseases. Food material generally include grains, vegetables, wild vegetables, edible fungi, fruits, poultry meat, livestock meat, eggs and milk, aquatic products, condiments and seasonings, etc. The following are some common food materials.

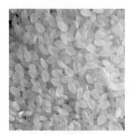

粳米 Polished round-grained rice

1. 粳米 Polished round-grained rice

【来源】为禾本科植物粳稻的种仁。

[Source] It is the seed kernel of japonica rice, a Gramineae plant.

【主要功用】可用于补养肠胃、止渴止泻。

[Functions] It can be used to nourish the stomach and the intestines, quench thirst and stop diarrhea.

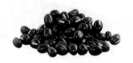

赤小豆 Adzuki beans

2. 赤小豆 Adzuki beans

【来源】为豆科植物赤小豆或赤豆的干燥成熟种子。

[Source] They are dried mature seeds of the Adzuki bean of the leguminous plant.

【主要功用】可用于治疗多种水肿、脚气、黄疸等疾病。

[Functions] Adzuki beans can be used to treat a variety of edema, beriberi, jaundice and other diseases.

3. 莲藕 Lotus root

【来源】为睡莲科植物莲的根茎的节部。

[Source] It is the nodal part of the rhizome of the Nymphaeaceae family.

【主要功用】可用于治疗热病、口渴、出血等。

[Functions] It can be used to treat fever, thirst, bleeding, etc.

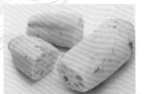

莲藕 Lotus root

4. 梨 Pear

【来源】为蔷薇科植物白梨、沙梨、秋子梨等栽培种的果实。

[Source] It is the fruit of cultivated species of the Rosaceae family, such as White pear, *Sha* pear, and *Qiuzi* pear.

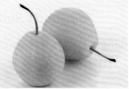

梨 Pear

【主要作用】可用于治疗热咳、少痰、咽干、心烦、口渴等。

[Functions] It can be used to treat hot cough, less sputum, dry throat, upset and thirst, etc.

三、经典药膳配方 Classic Medicinal Diet Formulas

（一）当归生姜羊肉汤 Chinese angelica, fresh ginger, and mutton soup

【组成】当归、生姜、羊肉。

[Composition] Chinese angelica , ginger , mutton.

【主要功用】适用于妇女产后气血虚弱，阳虚的腹痛、乳少，以及虚劳等。

[Functions] It is suitable for women with weak *qi*

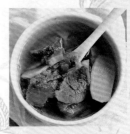

当归生姜羊肉汤
Chinese angelica, fresh ginger, and mutton soup

and blood after childbirth, abdominal pain, lack of breast milk, and fatigue.

【用法】取出当归、姜片，喝汤食肉。

[Usage] Take out Chinese angelica, ginger slice, drink soup and eat the mutton.

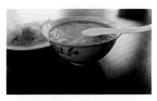

乌梅粥 Mume gruel

（二）乌梅粥 Mume gruel

【组成】乌梅、粳米、冰糖。

[Composition] Mume, polished round-grained rice, rock sugar.

【主要功用】适用于脾虚泄泻、痢疾、肺虚咳嗽、口渴等。

[Functions] Suitable for spleen deficiency diarrhea, dysentery, lung deficiency cough, thirst, etc.

【用法】空腹时温食。

[Usage] Eat warmly when the stomach is empty.

四、药膳制作方法举例 Example of How to Make Medicinal Diet

（一）茯苓造化糕的成分及功用 The ingredients and functions of Poria cocos cake

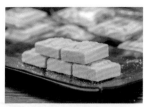

茯苓造化糕 Poria cocos cake

【组成】茯苓、莲子、山药、芡实、粳米、白糖。

[Composition] Poria cocos, lotus nut, Chinese yam, gordon euryale seed, polished round-grained rice, sugar.

【主要功用】补益脾胃，可用于改善脾胃虚弱、饮食不佳、泄泻等病症。

[Functions] It is used to nourish the spleen and the stomach, and it can be used for the weakness of the spleen and the stomach , poor diet, diarrhea and other diseases.

【用法】温食。

[Usage] Eat warmly.

（二）茯苓造化糕的制作流程 The preparation processes of Poria cocos cake

步骤一 食材准备。

Step 1 Food preparation.

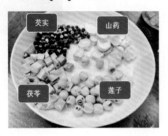
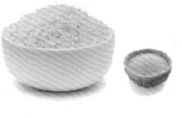

准备材料 Prepare materials

【食材】茯苓、莲子、山药、芡实各 10 克，粳米 1 000 克，白糖 500 克。

[Composition] 10 g of Poria cocos, lotus nuts, Chinese yam, gordon euryale seeds, 1,000 g of polished round-grained rice, 500 g of sugar.

步骤二 浸泡莲子。

Step 2 Soaking the lotus nuts.

莲子用温水浸泡，去皮，去芯。

Soak lotus nuts in warm water, peel and remove the core.

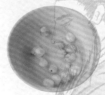

浸泡莲子 Soak lotus nuts

步骤三 磨成细粉。

Step 3 Grind into fine powder.

茯苓、莲子、山药、芡实、粳米、白糖混合在一起磨成细粉，放入盆内，加清水适量。

Mix Poria cocos, lotus nuts, Chinese yam, gordon

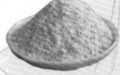

磨成细粉 Grind into fine powder

euryale seeds, polished round-grained rice, and sugar together, grind them into fine powder, and then put the powder into a basin with an appropriate amount of water.

步骤四　制作成型。

Step 4　Knead into shape.

把粉揉成面团，然后用模具制成蛋糕的形状。

Knead the powder into dough and then shape them into a cake.

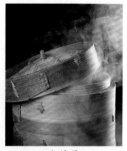

上笼蒸
Steam in a steamer
basket

步骤五　上笼蒸熟。

Step 5　Steam in a steamer.

把蛋糕蒸 20~30 分钟。

Steam the cake for 20–30 minutes.

任务分析 Task Analysis

1. 中药药膳的特点是什么？

What are the characteristics of Chinese medicinal diet?

_____

_____

2. 请说出几种药膳中常用的中药材原料。

Name several Chinese medicinal materials commonly used in medicinal diet.

_____

_____

3. 请说出几种药膳中常用的食物原料。

Name several food ingredients commonly used in medicinal diet.

_____

_____

4. 你知道今天制作了什么药膳吗？请说出这道药膳的主要成分和制作流程。

Do you know what medicinal diet has been prepared today? Please tell us the main ingredients and the preparation processes of this medicinal diet.

_____

_____

第三节　中药香囊

Section 3　Traditional Chinese Medicinal Sachets

根据香囊的制作方法，在中药调剂实训室制作中药香囊。

According to the method of making sachets, learn to make traditional Chinese medicinal sachets in the dispensing training room of Chinese materia medica.

学习目标　Learning Objectives

学会制作中药香囊。

To learn to make traditional Chinese medicinal sachets.

任务导入　Task Import

一、中药香囊的历史　The History of Traditional Chinese Medicinal Sachets

俗话说："戴个香草袋,不怕五虫害。"中药香囊又称"香包""香袋""荷包",在古代又被称为"衣冠疗法",将具有芳香辟秽功效的中药材装于衣帽、鞋袜或饰物中佩戴于身上，通过呼吸吸入或皮肤吸收从而发挥其防病治病的作用。

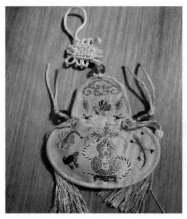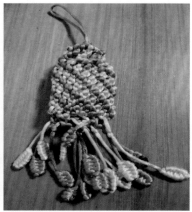

中药香囊
Traditional Chinese medicinal sachets

As the saying goes, when you wear a herbal bag, you will not be afraid of pests. Traditional Chinese medicinal sachets, which are known as sachets, sachet bags or sachet purses, and also called clothing therapy in ancient times, are used to play the role of disease prevention and treatment through breath inhalation or skin absorption by putting Chinese medicinal materials with the effect of aroma and avoiding pollution in clothes, hats, shoes, socks or accessories and wearing them on the body.

中药香囊的使用历史非常久远，早在先秦时期就有佩戴香囊的记载；到了近代，端午节期间中药香囊使用较为广泛，多用于驱恶避邪；现代，中医"治未病"的思想逐渐受到大家的重视，中药香囊的使用变得更加普遍，这里面也蕴含着丰富的中国传统文化底蕴和内涵。

The use of traditional Chinese medicinal sachets has a very long history. It was recorded to wear sachets as early as the pre-Qin period. In recent times, traditional Chinese medicinal sachets were widely used during the Dragon Boat Festival, which were mostly used to drive away evil spirits. In modern times, the thought of "treating the disease before its onset" in Traditional Chinese Medicine has gradually attracted everyone's attention, and the application of traditional Chinese medicinal sachets has become more common, which also contains rich traditional Chinese culture and connotation.

近年来，新冠疫情暴发，人类社会面临着疫情带来的重大威胁，中药香囊在抗疫中也发挥了非常重要的作用。

In recent years, with the outbreak of COVID-19, human society is facing severe challenges brought by the pandemics. Traditional Chinese medicinal sachets also play a very important role in the fight against pandemics.

二、用途和注意事项 Usage and Precautions of Traditional Chinese Medicinal Sachets

中药香囊一般具有多种用途，可用于节日祝愿、观赏品玩、疾病预防等多个方面，其中预防疾病为其最主要的用途。

Traditional Chinese medicinal sachets generally have a variety of applications, which can be used for festival wishes, ornamental products, disease prevention and so on, among which disease prevention is their most important usage.

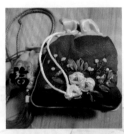

各式各样的中药香囊袋
All kinds of traditional Chinese medicinal sachets

中药香囊一年四季均可使用，但由于春夏秋冬气候特点不同，制作香囊的配方也不尽相同，预防的疾病也有所区别。香囊可随身佩戴或者悬挂于室内从而发挥相应的疗效。

Traditional Chinese medicinal sachets can be used all year round. The formulas of sachets made in different seasons are different.

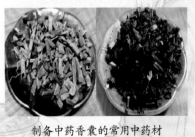

制备中药香囊的常用中药材
（藿香，紫苏）
Commonly used Chinese medicinal materials to prepare traditional Chinese medicinal sachets (Agastache rugosus, perilla)

As a result, the diseases to be prevented are different too. The sachets can be worn with people or hung indoors so as to give full play to their corresponding curative effect.

制备香囊所用的中药材一般均具芳香之性，现代医学认为这类中药材多含有挥发油，能产生独特的香气，这种香气可保护人体，使其免受病邪的侵袭。由于挥发油易挥发，所以中药香囊的香气一般只能持续 15~30 天，因此，香囊中的药物一般 7~15 天就需要更换一次。

Chinese medicinal materials used to prepare sachets generally possess aromatic characteristics, and modern medical world believes that this kind of Chinese medicinal materials mostly contain volatile oil and can produce unique aroma, which can protect human body from the invasion of pathogens. Because the volatile oil volatilize easily, the aroma of traditional Chinese medicinal sachets can only last for 15 to 30 days. Generally speaking, the medicinal materials in the sachets need to be replaced once every 7 to 15 days.

需要注意的是，并不是人人都适合使用中药香囊，过敏人群使用时须谨慎，应在医生指导下安全使用，孕妇、6 个月以下婴幼儿以及重症、急症患者不建议使用，对于儿童需特别注意，谨防其打开香囊出现误食现象。香囊虽好，使用须谨慎。

It should be noted that traditional Chinese medicinal sachets are not suitable for every people. They should be used safely with caution and under the guidance of doctors for people who are allergic to them. For pregnant women, children under 6 months and patients with severe emergencies, the sachets are not recommended. Special attention should be paid to children to prevent accidental eating when opening sachets. Although the sachets have good functions, be careful when using it.

三、常用功效的中药香囊配方 Formulas of Traditional Chinese Medicinal Sachets with Common Efficacy

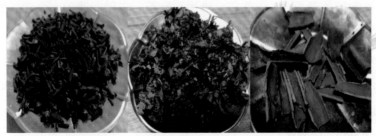

中药香囊配方中的常用中药材（丁香、艾叶、肉桂）

Commonly used Chinese medicinal materials in the formula of traditional Chinese medicinal Sachets（clove, folium artemisiae argyi, cinnamon）

儿童驱蚊香囊配方：艾叶、紫苏、金银花、丁香、藿香、薄荷、陈皮各8克，研成细粉，装入香囊。

Mosquito repellent formula for children is to take folium artemisiae argyi, purple perilla, honeysuckle, clove, Agastache rugosus, mint and dried tangerine peel 8g each, and grind them into fine powder and then put into a sachet.

成人预防感冒香囊配方：苍术、辛夷、川芎、白芷、藿香、羌活各8克，研成细粉，装入香囊。

Cold prevention formula for adults is to take rhizoma atractylodis, biond magnolia flowers, Szechuan lovage rhizome, radix angelicae, Agastache rugosus and incised notopterygium rhizome or root 8g each, and grind them into fine powder and then put into a sachet.

清心安神香囊配方：艾叶、紫苏、丁香、藿香、薄荷、陈皮、白芷、石菖蒲、金银花各5克，研成细粉，装入香囊。

Clearing heat and soothing the nerves formula is to take folium artemisiae argyi, purple perilla, clove, Agastache rugosus, mint, dried tangerine, radix angelicae, grassleaf sweetflag rhizome and honeysuckle 5g each, and grind them into fine powder and then put it into a sachet.

提神醒脑香囊配方：合欢花、佛手、薄荷、朱砂、琥珀、豆蔻、柏子仁、五味子各 2 克，研成细粉，装入香囊。

Refreshing the nerves and brain formula is to take albizia flower, finger citron mint, cinnabar, amber, round cardamon fruit, Chinese arborvitae kernel and Chinese magnoliavine fruit 2g each, and grind them into fine powder and then put it into a sachet.

四、中药香囊的制作过程 Preparation Process of Traditional Chinese Medicinal Sachets

（一）材料准备 Material preparation

准备制作中药香囊所需要用到的各种材料，主要为中药材、电子秤、粉碎机、香囊外袋、香囊内袋、PP 棉。

Prepare various materials for making traditional Chinese medicinal sachets, mainly including Chinese medicinal materials, electronic scale, grinder, outer sachet, inner sachet and PP cotton.

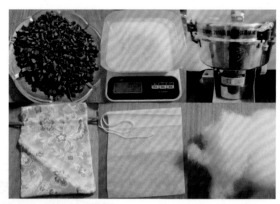

制作中药香囊所需要的材料（中药材、电子秤、粉碎机、香囊外袋、香囊内袋、PP 棉）
Materials required for preparing traditional Chinese medicinal sachets
（Chinese medicinal materials, electronic scale, grinder, outer sachet, inner sachet, PP cotton）

（二）制作过程 Making process of traditional Chinese medicinal sachets

下面我们以中药配方辛夷、川芎、白芷各8克为例，讲解中药香囊的制作。

Let's take the traditional Chinese medicinal formula of biond magnolia flowers, Szechuan lovage rhizome and radix angelicae 8g each as an example to explain the preparation processes of traditional Chinese medicinal sachets.

第一步，准备好所有的中药材。

The first step is to prepare all the Chinese medicinal materials.

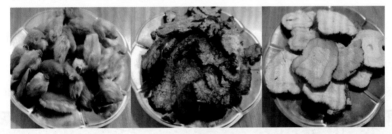

制备中药香囊所用的中药材（辛夷、川芎、白芷）
Chinese medicinal materials used to make traditional Chinese medicinal sachets
（biond magnolia flowers, Szechuan lovage rhizome, radix angelicae）

第二步，称取所需的每种中药材各8克。

The second step is to prepare 8g of each Chinese medicinal materials needed.

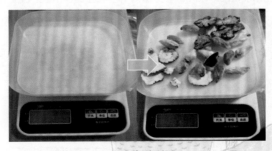

称量中药材
Weighing the Chinese medicinal materials

第三步，将中药材装入香囊内袋中。

The third step is to put the Chinese medicinal materials into the inner bag of a sachet.

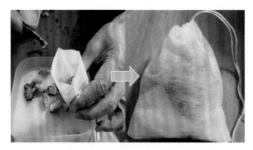

未粉碎的中药材直接装入香囊内袋
Put the uncrushed Chinese medicinal materials directly into the inner bag of a sachet

一种方法是将称好的中药材取适量直接装入香囊内袋中，束紧香囊内袋。

One method is to directly take an appropriate amount of the weighed Chinese medicinal materials and put them into the inner bag of a sachet and tighten the inner bag of the sachet.

另一种方法是将用粉碎机粉碎后的中药材细粉取适量装入香囊内袋中，束紧香囊内袋。

Another method is to crush the weighed Chinese medicinal materials into fine powder with a grinder and then put an appropriate amount of the fine powder into the inner bag of a sachet and tighten the inner bag of the sachet.

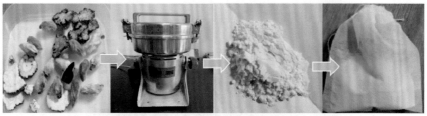

将中药材研磨成细粉后装入香囊内袋
Crush the Chinese medicinal materials into fine powder and then put into the inner bag of a sachet

第四步，将制作好的香囊内袋装入香囊外袋中，最终香囊制作完成。

The fourth step is to put the prepared inner bag of the sachet into the outer bag of the sachet, and finally the sachet is finished.

在这一步中，先将适量 PP 棉装入香囊外袋的底部，再装入第三步制作好的香囊内袋。香囊内袋装入后，再装入适量 PP 棉，整理香囊外袋的形状，并束紧香囊外袋，香囊制作完成。

First, put an appropriate amount of PP cotton into the bottom of the outer bag of the sachet, and then put the inner bag of the sachet made in the third step into the outer bag of the sachet. After filling the outer bag with the inner bag of the sachet, fill it again with an appropriate amount of PP cotton, and then sort out the shape of the outer bag of the sachet and tighten it. Finally the sachet is finished.

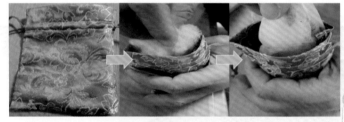

将 PP 棉和香囊内袋装入香囊外袋
Put PP cotton and the inner bag of the sachet into the outer bag of the sachet

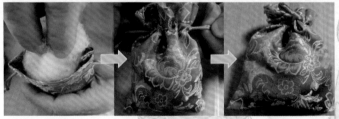

再次向香囊外袋中装入 PP 棉并整理香囊的外形
Put PP cotton again into the outer bag of the sachet and tidy the shape of it

任务分析 Task Analysis

1. 请判断孕妇是否可以使用以下配方的中药香囊。配方为檀香、小茴香各 3 克，丁香、辛夷各 15 克，冰片、麝香各少许。

Please judge whether the traditional Chinese medicinal sachet with the following formula can be used for pregnant women. The formula is 3g for each of sandalwood and fennel, 15g for each of clove and biond magnolia flowers, and a little of borneol and musk.

_____

_____

2. 请说出以丁香、艾叶各 5 克和肉桂 7.5 克为配方的驱蚊香囊的制作流程。

Please tell us the making processes of mosquito repellent sachet with 5g for each of clove and folium artemisiae argyi and 7.5g of cinnamon as the formula.

_____

_____

3. 请在图片下方写出制作中药香囊所用材料的名称。

Please write down the Chinese and English name of the materials used to make the traditional Chinese medicinal sachet below each picture.

①	②	③

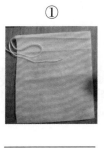 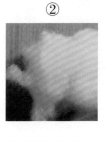 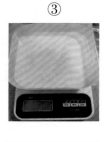

_____   _____   _____

_____   _____   _____

4. 请说出中药香囊有哪些用途。

Please name the applications of traditional Chinese medicinal sachets.

_____

_____

5. 请说出使用中药香囊时的注意事项。

Please state the cautions for using the traditional Chinese medicinal sachets.

_____

_____

6. 请判断以下哪些中药材可以用于制作中药香囊。

Please judge which of the following Chinese medicinal materials can be used to make sachets.

①红枣　　　　②藿香　　　　③甘草　　　　④草果

⑤八角茴香　　⑥黄芩

① Red dates　　　② Agastache rugosus　③ Licorice root

④ Amomum tsao-ko　⑤ Illicium verum　　⑥ Scutellaria baicalensis

_____

_____

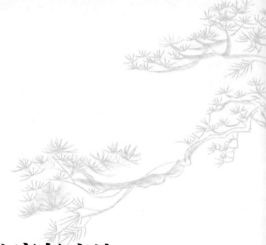

第四章　中国传统康复疗法

Chapter 4 Traditional Chinese Medical Rehabilitation

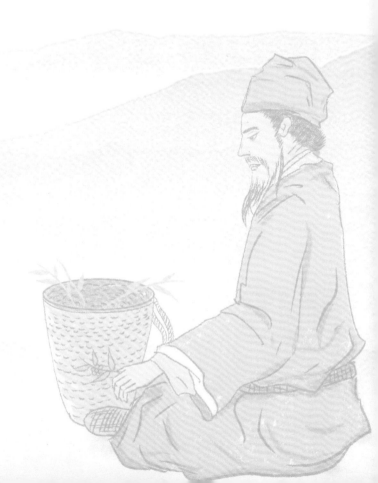

第一节 "神针" 之针刺疗法

Section 1 Magic Needles—Acupuncture

学习情境描述 Learning Situation Description

以教师示教、实践操作为主，以理论讲解为辅，在皮肤仿真模型上进行针刺手法练习，包括持针、进针、行针、出针等。

Based on teacher's demonstration and practical operation, supplemented by theoretical explanation, acupuncture manipulations are practiced on the skin simulation model, including needle holding, insertion, manipulation, and withdrawal.

学习目标 Learning Objectives

了解针刺疗法的起源，认识针刺工具，熟悉针刺操作的方法，掌握针刺疗法的注意事项。

To learn about the origin of acupuncture therapy, get to know acupuncture tools, be familiar with the methods of acupuncture manipulation, and master the precautions of acupuncture therapy.

任务导入 Task Import

针刺疗法，指利用金属制成的针具，通过一定的手法，刺激人体经络腧穴，从而防治疾病的治疗方法。

针刺疗法起源于中国，是一种非常古老的治病方法，有着数千年的悠久历史。在现代中国，仍然受到很多医生和患者的喜爱，在很多医院和诊所都能看见利用针灸来治疗疾病。

Acupuncture therapy refers to the use of metal needles through a certain manipulation to stimulate the human body's meridians and acupoints, so as to prevent and treat diseases.

Acupuncture therapy, originated in China, is a very ancient treatment method with a long history of thousands of years. In modern China, it is still popular with many doctors and patients, and the use of acupuncture can be seen in many hospitals and clinics to treat illnesses.

一、针具的演变 The Evolution of Needles

在远古时代，人们发生某些病痛不适的时候会不自觉地用手按摩、捶打，甚至用尖锐的石块按压疼痛不适的部位，人们发现这种做法能使原有的症状减轻或消失，因此最原始的针具——砭石出现了。砭石由石头制成，虽然足够锋利但并不尖锐，不能刺进皮肤，所以当时多用来切开皮肤、排脓放血或者按摩疼痛部位。随着社会生产力的不断发展，砭石逐渐发展成骨针、青铜针、铁针、金针、银针，直到现在所用的不锈钢针。除了材质不同以外，针具的形状构造也各不相同，在《黄帝内经·灵枢》中就记载了九种不同的针具，称为"九针"。由于形状不同，它们的作用也不尽相同。比如，尖锐的针可以刺入皮肤，圆钝的针可以按摩穴位，锋利的针可以切开皮肤而排脓放血。

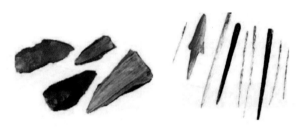

砭石 *Bian* stone

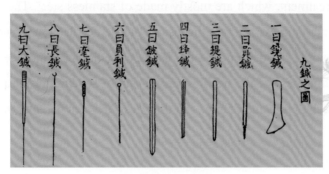

九针 The nine needles

In ancient times, when people had some pain or discomfort, they would unconsciously massage, beat with their hands, or even press the painful and uncomfortable parts with sharp stones to make the original symptoms lessen or disappear. Thus appeared the most primitive needle tool—*bian* stone. *Bian* stone is made of stone. Although it is very sharp, it can not pierce the skin. So it was mostly used to cut open the skin, drain pus, bleed or massage painful areas. With the continuous development of social productive forces, *bian* stone has gradually developed into bone needles, bronze needles, iron needles, gold needles, silver needles, and stainless steel needles used today. In addition to the material, the shape and structure of the needles are also different. Nine kinds of different needles are recorded in the *Huangdi Neijing·Lingshu*, which are called "Nine Needles". Because of their different shapes, they have different functions. For example, a sharp needle can pierce the skin, a round blunt needle can massage acupoints, and a keen-edged needle can cut the skin to drain pus and bleed.

在现代临床治疗中，最常用的针具是毫针，多由不锈钢制成，有良好的韧性和硬度，是一次性使用的无菌针具。其构造主要分成针柄、针身和针尖。毫针的长短粗细不一，通常我们会选择针身长度在 25~75 毫米，粗细在 0.32~0.38 毫米之间的针具。

Nowadays, the most commonly used needles are called filiform needles in clinical treatment, which are mostly made of stainless steel. They have good toughness and hardness, and are disposable sterile needles. The structure of the needles is mainly divided into needle handle, needle body and needle tip. The length and thickness of the needles vary. Usually, we choose the needles of a length between 25mm and 75mm, of a thickness between 0.32mm and 0.38mm.

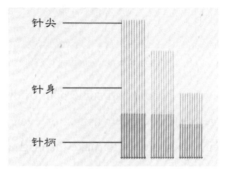

不同规格的毫针 Different sizes of filiform needles

二、针刺的操作程序 Acupuncture Procedure

为了完成针刺治疗，达到治病的目的，首先要掌握针刺的操作方法。其过程主要分为针刺前准备、针刺时操作和针刺后操作。

In order to achieve the goal of treating the disease with acupuncture, it is necessary to master the operation method of acupuncture. The process has three parts: the preparation before acupuncture, the operation during acupuncture and the operation after acupuncture.

（一）针刺前准备 The preparation before acupuncture

1. 体位的摆放 Body position

针刺治疗前应指导患者摆放合适的体位。体位的选择有三个原则：一是便于腧穴的定位，二是便于医者施术操作，三是让患者感觉舒适。临床常用体位以仰卧位、俯卧位、侧卧位和坐位为主。体位摆放好后，将患者的衣物拉起，充分暴露治疗部位，并且注意保暖。对精神紧张、体质虚弱的患者，应尽量采取卧位，以防病人感到疲劳或晕针。

Before acupuncture treatment, the patient should be instructed to lie a proper body position. There are three principles for the selection of body positions: ① to facilitate the positioning of acupoints, ② to facilitate the operation of the doctor, and ③ to make the patient feel comfortable. The most commonly used positions are supine, prone, lateral and sitting. After the body position is set, the doctor has to pull up the patient's clothing to expose the treatment area and then keep warm. For nervous and weak patients, the supine position should be taken as much as possible to prevent the patient from feeling fatigued or fainting.

2. 定穴 Find the correct acupoints

定穴，即找到正确的针刺部位。腧穴的定位准确与否直接关系到针刺的疗效。为了保证定穴的准确性，可在针刺前用手指按压该部位，一般出现比较明显的局部酸胀感即为腧穴所在之处。

Whether the acupoints are accurately located is directly related to the efficacy of acupuncture. In order to locate the acupoint accurately, the doctor can press the area with fingers before acupuncture. Generally, there is an obvious local sour swelling sensation when the acupoint is pressed.

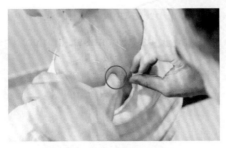

定穴 Find the correct acupoints

3. 针刺前消毒 Disinfection before acupuncture

现在所用的工具是一次性无菌针灸针，可以直接使用，无须消毒。但医生手指和针刺部位的消毒必不可少。针刺治疗前，医生应先用肥皂水将手洗干净，擦拭干后用75%酒精棉球涂擦手指指腹才可持针。最后在针刺部位用75%酒精棉球从进针部位的中心向外绕圈擦拭。已消毒的皮肤应防止重新污染。

The tools used now are disposable sterile acupuncture needles, which can be used directly without disinfection. However, disinfection of the doctor's fingers and the patient's skin is necessary. Before acupuncture, the doctor should wash hands with soap, and then use 75% alcohol cotton balls to rub the fingers before holding the needle. Finally, use a 75% alcohol cotton ball to wipe the acupuncture site outwards from the center of the needle insertion site. Disinfected skin should be protected from re-contamination.

（二）针刺时操作 The operation during acupuncture

1. 持针和进针 Holding and inserting the needle

以右利手为例，先用右手的二指捏住针柄靠下的位置，中指或无名指指端紧靠穴位，指腹抵住针身下段，然后捏住针柄的手指向下用力，即可将针刺入皮肤。最后继续将针向下刺入合适的深度方可停止。

Taking the right-handedness as an example, firstly use two or three fingers to pinch the lower part of the needle handle, and then put the middle finger or the ring finger close to the acupoint, with the pulp of the finger against the lower part of the needle body. Then press down with the fingers holding the needle handle to pierce into the skin. Finally, continue to pierce the needle down to an appropriate depth.

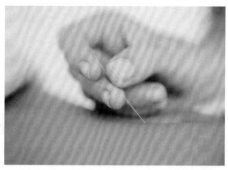

持针姿势 The posture of holding the needle

2. 行针 Manipulating the needle

为了取得更好的疗效，针刺入皮肤后还需实施行针的操作。行针的方法分为两种：提插和捻转。

In order to get a better effect, after the needle is pierced into the skin, there are two methods for manipulating the needles: lifting-thrusting and twirling.

提插是用手指捏住针柄将针体做上提、下插的运动。捻转是顺时针、逆时针交替地转动针柄。提插和捻转的目的是让针刺部位产生酸、麻、胀等异常感觉，这样才能获得更好的治疗效果。

Lifting and thrusting is the upward and downward movement of the needle body by pinching the needle handle with fingers. Twirling is turning the needle handle clockwise and counterclockwise. The purpose of lifting and thrusting and twirling is to make the acupuncture part produce abnormal sensations such as soreness, numbness, swelling, etc, so as to have a better therapeutic effect.

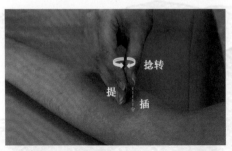

提插和捻转 Lifting and thrusting and twirling

3. 留针 Retaining the needle

毫针刺入腧穴后，不会被立即取出，而是要停留一段时间，一般在10~30分钟。留针是为了加强针刺感应，保证针刺刺激的时间，以此加强治疗效果。留针过程中可反复行针，以获得更好的效果。

After the filiform needle is inserted into the acupoint, it will not be taken out immediately, but stay for a period of time, usually 10–30 minutes. The purpose of retaining the needle is to strengthen the induction of acupuncture and ensure the time for acupuncture stimulation. This enhances the therapeutic effect. Needle retention can be repeated for better results. In the process of needle retention, repeated needling manipulation can get a better effect.

在留针期间，应注意患者的面色和表情，观察其是否出现疲劳、头晕、恶心、心慌、面色苍白、出汗等现象。一旦出现，应立即将针取出，协助患者静卧，给以温水，注意保暖，通常患者休息片刻即可恢复。

During the needle retention, the doctor should pay attention to the patient's complexion and expression. If the patient has fatigue, dizziness, nausea, palpitation, pale complexion, sweating and other symptoms, the needle should be taken out immediately. And the patient should lie down, drink warm water, and keep warm. He will recover after a short rest.

4. 出针 Withdrawing the needle

治疗结束后，需要将所有针全部取出。为了减少因局部出血而出现的血肿，一般先用左手持消毒干棉球按住针孔周围的皮肤，右手持针轻微捻转，慢慢将针提至皮下，然后将针拔出。出针后轻压针孔片刻再将干棉球移开，以防出血。

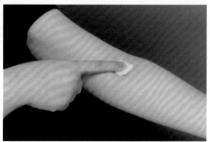

按压针孔　Press the needle hole after withdrawing the needle

At the end of the treatment, all needles need to be removed. In order to reduce the risk of hematoma caused by local bleeding, the doctor will hold a sterile dry cotton ball in the left hand to press the skin slightly on the acupoint, twirl the needle slightly with the right hand, lift the needle slowly to the subcutaneous, and then pull it out. After the needle has been removed, the dry cotton ball can be removed after a few moments of gentle pressure on the needle hole to prevent bleeding.

三、针刺的注意事项 Cautions for Acupuncture

患者过于饥饿、疲劳、精神过度紧张时，不宜立即进行针刺。应尽可能选用卧位。

Acupuncture should not be used immediately when the patient is too hungry, fatigued, or nervous. The supine position should be used whenever possible.

不宜针刺孕妇的小腹部和腰部。

Acupuncture should not be used in the lower abdomen and waist of pregnant women.

婴儿在囟门未闭合时，头顶部的腧穴不宜针刺。

Acupuncture should not be used in the unclosed fontanelle area of infants.

皮肤有感染、溃疡、瘢痕或肿瘤的部位，不宜针刺。

Acupuncture should not be used on infection, ulcer, scar or tumor on the skin.

对患有出血性疾病、有自发性出血或损伤后出血不止的患者，不宜针刺。

Acupuncture is not suitable for patients with bleeding disorders, spontaneous bleeding or persistent bleeding after injury.

针刺深度不宜过深以防刺破内脏。

Do not insert the needles too deep in skin, or it may puncture the internal organs.

如出针困难勿要强行拔针。

The needle should not be taken out forcefully if it is difficult to withdraw.

如果出现晕针，应立即停止针刺，拔针，使患者平卧休息，予服温开水或糖水，即可恢复。

In case of needle fainting, stop acupuncture and pull out the needles immediately, make the patient lie flat and rest, and take warm boiled water or sugar water for recovery.

任务分析 Task Analysis

1. 辨别最早的砭石以及现在常用的毫针。

Identify the earliest *bian* stones and the filiform needles commonly used today.

_____

_____

2. 思考治疗前应如何指导患者的体位摆放。

Think about how to guide the patient into a right body position before treatment.

_____

_____

3. 说出并完成针刺操作前的消毒步骤。

Tell and complete the disinfection steps before inserting the needle.

_____

_____

4. 完成持针、进针、行针、出针的操作。

Complete the operation of needle holding, insertion, manipulation and withdrawal.

_____

_____

第二节 "香火"之灸法

Section 2 Aromatous Fire—Moxibustion

学习情境描述 Learning Situation Description

以教师示教、实践操作为主，理论讲解为辅，学习灸法的相关知识。

To learn about moxibustion based on teacher's demonstration and practical operation, supplemented by theoretical explanation.

学习目标 Learning Objectives

了解灸法诞生的历史，认识施灸的材料，掌握各种施灸的方法，掌握施灸的注意事项。

To know the history of the birth of moxibustion and the material of moxibustion, master various methods of moxibustion, and the cautions of moxibustion.

任务导入 Task Import

上一节我们介绍了针刺疗法，除此之外，还有一种中医疗法同样具有悠久的历史，我们称为"灸法"。由于操作步骤简单，灸法成了家庭常见的保健方法，深受人们的喜爱。

In the previous section, acupuncture therapy is introduced. In addition to this, there is another traditional Chinese therapy with a long history, which is called moxibustion therapy. Because of the simple operation steps, moxibustion therapy has become a common method of home health care and is deeply loved by people.

一、灸法的起源 The Origin of Moxibustion

说到灸法的起源，不得不提到人类对火的使用。在远古时代，学会了使用火的古人发现用火适当熏烤或烧灼身体的某些部位，能够减轻甚至治愈病痛。这就是灸法的诞生。

When it comes to the origin of moxibustion, we have to mention the use of fire by humans. In ancient times, people who had learned how to use fire found that roasting or burning certain parts of the body with fire could relieve or even recover from the pain. This is the origin of moxibustion.

后来，又经过不断实践，古人尝试了很多能燃烧的材料，如松、柏、桑、槐等，但因为对人体有所伤害，它们都逐渐被淘汰下来。最终，易燃、安全、有效的艾草被选为灸法的主要材料。

Later, after continuous practice, the ancients tried many kinds of combustible materials, such as pine, cypress, mulberry, locust, etc., but they were gradually eliminated because of the harm to the human body. Finally, flammable, safe and effective wormwood was selected as the main material of moxibustion.

二、艾灸的材料 The Materials of Moxibustion

（一）艾草 Wormwood

艾草是如今最常见的灸法药材。《本草纲目》记载，艾草味苦、辛，性温，归脾、肝、肾经。气味芳香，易燃，有温通经络、散寒止痛、保健强身的功效。

Today wormwood is the most common medicinal materials in moxibustion. *The Grand Compendium of Materia Medica* records: wormwood is bitter, acrid, warm in nature, and takes effect to the spleen, the liver and the kidney meridians. The flammable materials smell fragrant, and have the functions of warming the meridians, dispelling cold, relieving pain, and keeping health.

长期医疗实践证明，艾草是最好的灸法原料。因为它燃烧时火力持久温和，穿透力强，安全又经济，有很好的药用价值。

It is proved that wormwood is the best medicinal material for moxibustion therapy, because it burns with lasting and mild fire. The heat can be transformed deep into the skin and muscle. It is safe, cheap, and valuable.

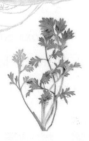

艾草 Wormwood

（二）艾绒 Moxa wool

新鲜的艾草经过一定程序的加工后才能使用，我们把成品称为"艾绒"。艾绒是怎么制成的呢？先要把艾草经过反复曝晒、捶打、捣碎，再去除其中的杂质，最终形成软细的绒状物，这就是艾绒。艾绒的质量有好坏之分，时间越久、越纯净的艾绒质量越好，三年以上的陈艾最好。

Moxa wool is made of fresh wormwood. How is it made? Firstly, the wormwood must be repeatedly exposed to the sun, beaten, and mashed, and then the impurities are removed, and finally the wormwood turns into moxa wool. The quality of moxa wool is different.The pure moxa wool which is kept for a long time is much better. The moxa wool that is kept for more than three years is the best.

（三）艾炷和艾条 Moxa cone and moxa stick

施行灸法之前我们还要把艾绒做成不同的形状，一般为两种：艾炷和艾条。

Moxa wool is generally made into two different shapes: the moxa cone and the moxa stick.

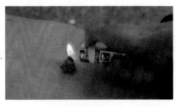

艾炷 Moxa cone

艾炷是将纯净的艾绒用手搓捏成圆锥形的艾团。艾炷有大、中、小之分，大小如蚕豆者为大炷，如黄豆者为中炷，如麦粒者为小炷。施灸时以艾炷的大小和壮数来控制刺激量。

The moxa cone is made of pure moxa wool, kneaded into a cone shape by hand. There are large, medium and small moxa cones. The size and number of moxa cones are used to control the amount of stimulation.

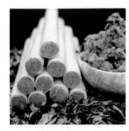

艾条 Moxa stick

艾条是用桑皮纸将艾绒包裹，卷成直径约 1.5 厘米、长约 20 厘米的圆柱状。

The moxa stick is made by wrapping moxa wool with mulberry paper and rolling it into a cylindrical shape with a diameter of about 1.5cm and a length of about 20cm.

三、艾灸的用法 The Use of Moxibustion

根据操作方法的不同分为艾炷灸、艾条灸、温针灸和温灸器灸。

According to the different operation methods, moxibustion is divided into moxa cone moxibustion, moxa stick moxibustion, warming needle moxibustion and moxa burner moxibustion.

（一）艾炷灸 Moxa cone moxibustion

1. 直接灸 Direct moxibustion

直接灸是将艾炷直接放在皮肤上进行燃烧。

Direct moxibustion: Put the burning moxa cone directly on the skin.

2. 间接灸 Indirect moxibustion

间接灸是用间隔物将皮肤和艾炷分隔开。作为间隔物的材料有很多种，如生姜、食盐、大蒜等。

Indirect moxibustion uses other materials to separate the skin from the moxa cone. Many materials can be used to separate the skin and the moxa cone, such as ginger, salt, garlic, etc.

常见的间接灸有以下三种：There are 3 kinds of common indirect moxibustion：

（1）隔姜灸 Ginger-separated moxibustion

取直径 2~3 厘米、厚约 0.5 厘米的生姜一片，用针在姜片上刺数孔，放上艾炷，再将姜片放在治疗部位上，最后点燃。此法可治疗感冒、呕吐、腹痛、泄泻、关节疼痛、遗精、阳痿、痛经等。

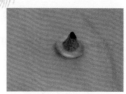

隔姜灸 Ginger-separated moxibustion

Take a piece of ginger about 2–3 cm in diameter and 0.5 cm in thickness, prick several holes in the ginger with a needle, place a moxa cone on it, then place the ginger on the treatment area and finally light the moxa cone. This method can treat colds, vomiting, abdominal pain, diarrhea, joint pain, nocturnal emission, impotence, dysmenorrhea, etc.

（2）隔蒜灸 Garlic-seperated moxibustion

把大蒜头切成厚约 0.5 厘米的薄片，以针刺数孔，放在穴位处，然后将艾炷放在蒜片上，点燃施灸。本法多用于治疗瘰疬、肺痨及初起的肿疡等症。

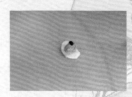

隔蒜灸 Garlic-separated moxibustion

Slice garlic into pieces about 0.5 cm in thickness, and then prick holes in it. A slice of garlic should be placed on the acupoint with the moxa cone on it and light the cone. This method is mostly used for the treatment of scrofula, tuberculosis and early-onset ulcers.

（3）隔盐灸 Salt-separated moxibustion

先用纯净的食盐将脐部填满，再放上一个薄姜片，上置大艾炷，用火

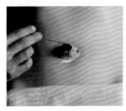

隔盐灸 Salt-separated
moxibustion

点燃。本法有回阳、救逆、固脱的功效，但必须连续治疗，直到症状改善。多用于治疗虚劳证等。

First fill the umbilicus with pure salt, and then put a thin slice of ginger, with a large moxa stick on it. This method has the effect of returning *yang*, stemming counterflow and desertion, but it must be treated continuously until the symptoms are improved. It is mostly used for the treatment of deficiency-consumption and so on.

（二）艾条灸 Moxa stick moxibustion

艾条灸的方法较为简单，易于掌握，分为悬起灸和实按灸两种，以前者最为常见。

The method of moxa stick moxibustion is relatively simple and easy to master. It is divided into two types: suspended moxibustion and pressing moxibustion. The former is the most common.

（三）温针灸 Warming needle moxibustion

温针灸是将针刺和艾灸结合的一种方法，适用于既需要留针又需要施灸的病症。操作方法是，针刺入腧穴得气后，用一段长约2厘米左右的艾条，插在针柄上，点燃施灸。这样能使热力通过针身传入体内，达到治疗目的。

Warming needle moxibustion is a method that combines acupuncture and moxibustion. It is suitable for patients who require both needle retention and moxibustion. The operation method is that after the needle is inserted into the acupoint to obtain *qi* , a moxa stick about 2 cm long is inserted onto the needle handle and the stick is ignited. In this way, heat can be transferred into the body through the needle to achieve the purpose of treatment.

（四）温灸器灸 Moxa burner moxibustion

现在常见的温灸器是木质的长方形或正方形盒，上方有孔，下方是金属丝网。将艾条点燃后从上孔插入，调整到合适的高度后放在需要施灸的部位，直到所灸部位的皮肤变得红润。这种方法对小儿、妇女及害怕灸法的人最为适宜。

Now the common device is a wooden rectangular or square box with holes above and a wire mesh below. Ignite the moxa sticks, insert them from the upper hole of the box and adjust the moxa sticks to a suitable height. Put the box on the body part needed to be treated until the skin is rosy. This method is suitable for children, women and people who are afraid of moxibustion.

四、灸后调复 Rehabilitation after Moxibustion Treatment

灸法治疗结束后，患者应休息片刻。治疗后局部毛孔打开，要注意防寒、保暖、避风，多喝温水，并且2小时内不要洗澡，切忌凉水洗浴。

After moxibustion treatment, the patient needs to rest for a while. While the local pores are opened, the patient should keep warm, shelter from the wind, and drink some warm water. Do not take a bath within 2 hours, and avoid taking a bath with cold water.

五、注意事项 Cautions for Moxibustion

头面五官、乳头、大血管经过处、关节处等部位不宜使用直接灸，以免烫伤。

It is not advisable to use direct moxibustion on the head, face, nipples, locations that large blood vessels pass through, and joints to avoid burning.

妊娠期妇女的腰骶部、下腹部不宜使用灸法。

Moxibustion treatment should not be used on the waist and lower abdomen of pregnant women.

极度疲劳、饥饿、饱腹、酒醉、大汗淋漓状态下或妇女经期不宜使用灸法。

Under the condition of extreme fatigue, hunger, full stomach, drunkenness, sweating profusely or women's menstrual period, moxibustion should not be used.

对于身体虚弱的患者，治疗时艾炷不宜过大，刺激量不宜过强，以防晕灸。一旦出现晕灸，应立即停止治疗，并让患者躺下静卧片刻。

For weak patients, the moxa cone should not be too large and the stimulation should not be too strong during the treatment to prevent dizziness. Once dizziness occurs, the treatment should be stopped immediately, and the patient should lie down for a while.

灸法治疗过程中要防止燃烧的艾绒脱落，烧伤皮肤或损坏衣物。

In the course of moxibustion treatment, the burning moxa wool must be prevented from falling off, burning the skin or damaging the clothing.

任务分析 Task Analysis

1. 说出使用艾草作为灸法材料的原因。

Talk about the reason for using wormwood as a moxibustion material.

_____

_____

2. 学习如何制作艾炷。

Learn how to make moxa cones.

_____

_____

3. 完成各种灸法的操作，如直接灸、间接灸、艾条灸、温针灸等。

Practice various moxibustion methods, such as direct moxibustion, indirect moxibustion, moxa stick moxibustion, warming needle moxibustion, etc.

_____

_____

4. 分析灸法操作时的注意事项。

Analyze the cautions in moxibustion operation.

_____

_____

第三节 "妙手" 之按摩点穴

Section 3 Skillful Hand-massage and Acupoint Pressing

学习情境描述 Learning Situation Description

根据经络学说和按摩手法，进行自我保健按摩操作。

According to the meridian-collateral theory and massage techniques, carry out self-care massage operation.

学习目标 Learning Objectives

能够运用按摩技术进行常见疾病的保健预防。

To be able to use massage skills for health-care and prevention of common diseases.

任务导入 Task Import

一、认识经络腧穴 Understanding Meridians and Acupoints

经络是经脉和络脉的总称。人体经络包括点、线、面三个部分。所谓点，除了 360 多个经穴之外，还有很多奇穴，另有天应穴、不定穴等，所谓"人身寸寸皆是穴"，其数不可胜数。至于线，有正脉、支脉、别脉、络脉、孙脉、奇脉、经隧等各种纵横交错和深浅密布的循行径路。至于面，肢体的皮肉筋骨和脏腑组织都有一般的分布和特殊的联系。

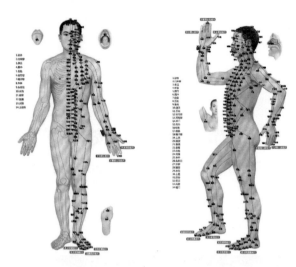

经络腧穴 Meridians and acupoints

Meridians are the general name of meridians and collaterals. The meridians and collaterals of the human body include points, lines and areas. In addition to more than 360 meridians points, there are many extra points, as well as aishi points. As the saying goes, "every inch of the human body is an acupoint." The number of the point is innumerable. As for the line, there are all kinds of crisscrossing and densely distributed paths, such as the main, branch, other, *luo*, *sun*, odd and meridian channels. As for the area, the flesh, muscles, bones of the limbs and tissues of *zang-fu* organs all have general distribution and special connection.

经络不像心脏、肝脏、血管、四肢等是看得见的，而是人体内部遵循一定线路、互相联系、沟通内外、传输气血的隐性系统，解剖时看不见，但遇到情况人体却能有所感觉。形象地说，人体就像一座城市，而经络就如同城市中的各种管道。在这些管道中，大的主干叫经脉，小的分支叫络脉。它们纵横交错，遍布全身，向内连接着人体的五脏六腑，向外沟通着人体的四肢百骸、五官九窍。总之，经络将人体各部分组织器官联系成为一个富有生机和活力的有机整体。

Unlike the heart, the liver, the blood vessels, the limbs and so on, meridians are invisible but a hidden system that follows a certain line, connects with each other, communicates the inside and the outside, and transmits blood and *qi* inside the human body. It can't be seen by anatomy, but the human body can feel it in case of situation. Figuratively speaking, the human body is like a city, and the meridians are like various pipelines in the city. Among these pipelines, the larger trunks are called meridians and the smaller branches are called collaterals. They crisscross all over the body, connecting the internal organs of the human body inward and communicating all the limbs and bones, five sense organs and nine orifices of the human body outward. In short, the meridians connect the tissues and organs of various parts of the human body into a vibrant and dynamic organic whole.

穴位是中医学独有的名词，指人体经络线上特殊的点区部位。穴位又称"腧穴"，负责人体脏腑经络气血的输注和出入。穴位并非孤立的存在，而是与人体内部的各组织器官存在密切的联系。一般而言，穴位由内而外能够反映病痛，由外而内则可通过刺激来防治疾病。正因为如此，中医常常将穴位作为疾病的反应点和治疗的刺激点，通过针刺、推拿、点按、艾灸等方法刺激相应的穴位，对症治病。

Acupoint is a unique term in Traditional Chinese Medicine, which refers to a special point area on the meridian line of the human body. Acupoints, also known as "Shuxue" in Chinese, are responsible for the infusion and access of *qi* and blood in the internal organs, meridians and collaterals of the human body. Acupoints are not isolated, but closely related to various tissues and organs in the human body. Generally speaking, they can be stimulated from the inside out to respond to illness and pain, and from the outside in to prevent and treat diseases. Because of this, Traditional Chinese Medicine often takes acupoints as the reaction point of diseases and the stimulation point of treatment, and stimulates the corresponding acupoints through acupuncture, *tuina*, pointing, pressing, moxibustion and other methods to treat diseases.

二、常见腧穴介绍 Introduction to Common Acupoints

（一）头面颈项部腧穴 Acupoints on head, face and neck

1. 百会（GV20）Baihui

【定位】在头部，两耳尖与头正中线相交处。

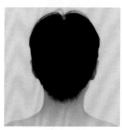

百会（GV20）Baihui

【Location】At the junction of a line connecting the apices of the ears and the midline of the head.

【主治】头部保健重要穴位，可治疗头痛、眩晕、失眠、脑梗后遗症等。

【Indications】It is an important acupoint for head health care, which can treat headache, dizziness, insomnia, sequelae of cerebral infarction, etc.

2. 四白（ST2）Sibai

【定位】在面部，目正视，瞳孔直下，当眶下孔凹陷处。

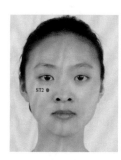

四白（ST2）Sibai

【Location】On the face, with the eyes looking straight ahead, directly below the centre of the pupil, in the depression at the infraorbital foramen.

【主治】按摩该穴既防眼病又具美容功效，可以预防皱纹、改善皮肤，还可治疗目赤肿痛、眼睑眴动、口眼歪斜、近视、色盲等。

【Indications】Massaging this point not only prevents eye diseases, but also has a cosmetic effect. Massaging Sibai acupoints can prevent wrinkles and improve skin condition. It can also treat sore red swollen eyes, eyelid movement, deviated eyes and mouth, myopia, color blindness and so on.

3. 睛明（BL1）Jingming

【定位】在面部，目内眦内上方眶内侧壁凹陷中。

【Location】On the face, it's located in a depression superior and medial to the inner canthus of the eye.

【主治】主治目赤肿痛、近视等眼科疾病和急性腰扭伤等。

【Indications】It mainly treats eye diseases such as sorered swollen eyes, myopia and so on, and acute lumbar sprain, etc.

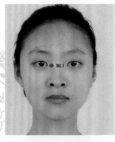

睛明（BL1）Jingming

4. 迎香（LI20）Yingxiang

【定位】在鼻翼外缘中点旁，鼻唇沟中。

【Location】Near the midpoint of the outer edge of the nasal wing, in the nasolabial groove.

【主治】按摩此穴具有通经活络、通利鼻窍的作用，常用于治疗鼻塞、嗅觉减退、急慢性鼻炎、面瘫、胆道蛔虫症等。

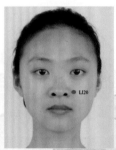

迎香（LI20）
Yingxiang

【Indications】Massaging this point has the functions of dredging meridians and activating collaterals, and clearing nasal orifices. It is commonly used to treat nasal congestion, anosmia, acute and chronic rhinitis, facial paralysis, biliary ascariasis, etc.

5. 太阳（EX-HN5）Taiyang

【定位】在头部，眉梢与目外眦之间，向后约一横指的凹陷中。

【Location】On the temple, in a depression approximately one horizontal finger lateral to the midpoint of a line connecting the lateral extremity of the eyebrow

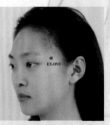

太阳（EX-HN5）
Taiyang

and the outer canthus of the eye.

【主治】目赤肿痛、眼睛干涩、头痛、牙痛、口眼㖞斜。

【Indications】Sore red swollen eyes, dry eyes, headache, toothache, facial paralysis.

6. 风池（GB20）Fengchi

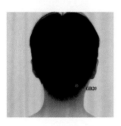

风池（GB20）
Fengchi

【定位】在颈后区，枕骨之下，胸锁乳突肌上端与斜方肌上端之间的凹陷中。

【Location】At the lower border of the occipital bone, in the depression between the upper end of sternocleidomastoid muscle and the upper end of trapezius muscle.

【主治】头痛、失眠、癫痫、颈部疼痛、感冒、鼻塞、耳鸣等。

【Indications】Headache, insomnia, epilepsy, neck pain, cold, nasal congestion, tinnitus, etc.

7. 大椎（DU14）Dazhui

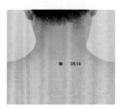

大椎（DU14）
Dazhui

【定位】在脊柱区，第七颈椎棘突下凹陷中，后正中线上。

【Location】In the spinal region, in the depression below the spinous process of the 7th cervical vertebra on the posterior midline.

【主治】感冒、发热、咳嗽、头痛、颈部不适等。

【Indications】Cold, fever, cough, headache, neck discomfort, etc.

（二）胸腹部腧穴 Acupoints on chest and abdomen

1. 关元（CV4）Guanyuan

【定位】在下腹部，脐中下 3 寸，前正中线上。（将脐中与耻骨联合上

缘中点的连线平分为 5 等份，该连线的上 3/5 与下 2/5 交点处即为本穴）

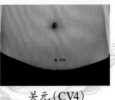

关元（CV4）
Guanyuan

【Location】In the lower abdomen, 3 *cun* inferior to the umbilicus on the anterior midline. (Divide the connecting line between the centre of umbilicus and the midpoint of the upper edge of pubic symphysis into 5 equal parts, and the intersection of the upper 3/5 and the lower 2/5 of the connecting line is this point)

【主治】该穴为保健强壮的要穴。长期刺激关元穴对于各种虚损性病症及泌尿生殖系统病症有很好的疗效。

【Indications】It is an important point for health care and strength. Long-term stimulation of Guanyuan point has a good curative effect on various asthenic diseases and diseases of urogenital system.

2. 气海（CV6）Qihai

【定位】在下腹部，脐中下 1.5 寸，前正中线上。（仰卧位或正坐位，从肚脐起沿下腹部前正中线直下 2 横指，食中二指并拢，以中指近端指间关节横纹水平的二指宽度为 1.5 寸）

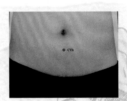

气海（CV6）Qihai

【Location】In the lower abdomen, 1.5 *cun* inferior to the umbilicus on the anterior midline. (In the supine or sitting position, the lower two horizontal fingers are straight along the front midline of the lower abdomen from the navel, the middle two fingers are close together, and the width of the two fingers at the level of the transverse line of the proximal interphalangeal joint of the middle finger is 1.5 *cun*)

【主治】此穴为保健强壮要穴。按摩气海穴可防治中风脱证、乏力、腹痛、泄泻、痢疾、便秘、小便不利、遗尿、遗精、阳痿、月经不调、崩漏、水肿、气喘等。

【Indications】This is an important acupoint for health care and strengthening. Massaging Qihai can prevent and treat stroke desertion pattern, fatigue, abdominal pain, diarrhea, dysentery, constipation, adverse urination, enuresis, spermatorrhea, impotence, irregular menstruation, metrorrhagia, edema, asthma, etc.

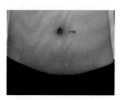

神阙（CV8）Shenque

3. 神阙（CV8）Shenque

【定位】在脐区，脐中央。

【Location】In the center of umbilicus.

【主治】按摩该穴对腹痛肠鸣、泄泻、痢疾、便秘、脱肛、水肿、小便不利等有独特疗效。

【Indications】Massaging this acupoint has a unique curative effect on abdominal pain, rumbling intestines, diarrhea, dysentery, constipation, anal prolapse, edema, adverse urination and so on.

（三）上肢部腧穴 Acupoints on upper limbs

1. 合谷（LI4）Hegu

【定位】在手背，第1、2掌骨间，第2掌骨桡侧中点处。

【Location】On the back of the hand, between the first and the second metacarpal bones, and at the midpoint of the radial side of the second metacarpal bone.

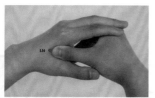

合谷（LI4）Hegu

【主治】治疗头面部疾病首选穴位。可治疗头痛、眩晕、目赤肿痛、咽喉肿痛、齿痛、口眼㖞斜、鼻出血、腹痛、便秘等。

【Indications】Hegu is the first choice for the treatment of head and face diseases. It can be used to treat headache, dizziness, sore red swollen eyes, sore throat, toothache, deviated eyes and mouth, nosebleed, abdominal pain, constipation, etc.

2. 内关（PC6）Neiguan

【定位】在前臂前区，腕掌侧远端横纹上2寸，掌长肌腱与桡侧腕屈肌腱之间。

【Location】In the forearm anterior area, 2 *cun* above the transverse stria of the distal carpometacarpal side, between the palmaris longus tendon and the radial wrist flexor tendon.

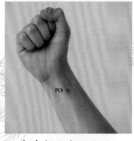

内关（PC6）Neiguan

【主治】按摩该穴对心悸、胸闷、心动过速或过缓、心律不齐、冠心病、心绞痛等都有疗效，还能防止晕车、晕船。

【Indications】Massaging this acupoint is effective for palpitation, chest tightness, tachycardia or bradycardia, arrhythmia, coronary heart disease, angina pectoris, and can also prevent carsickness and seasickness.

3. 曲池（LI11）Quchi

【定位】在肘区，屈肘成直角，在肘横纹外侧端与肱骨外上髁连线中点处。

【Location】In the elbow area, flex the elbow at 90° approximately, at the midpoint of the line

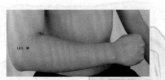

曲池（LI11）Quchi

between the lateral end of the transverse pattern of the elbow and the lateral epicondyle of the humerus.

【主治】肩肘关节痛、发热、头痛、眩晕、腹痛、湿疹等。

【Indications】Shoulder and elbow pain, fever, headache, dizziness, abdominal pain, eczema, etc.

（四）下肢部腧穴 Acupoints on lower limbs

1. 足三里（ST36）Zusanli

【定位】在小腿外侧，髌韧带外侧凹陷下3寸，胫骨前嵴外1横指。

【Location】On the outside of the leg, 3 *cun* below the lateral depression

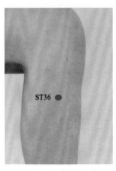

足三里（ST36）
Zusanli

of the patellar ligament, and 1 transverse finger outside the crest of the anterior tibial muscle.

【主治】按摩该穴可提高人体免疫力。经常按摩足三里可治疗胃痛、恶心、消化不良、便秘、腹泻、头痛、眩晕、失眠、心悸气短、乳腺炎等。

【Indications】Massaging this point can improve human immunity. Regular massage of Zusanli can treat stomach pain, nausea, dyspepsia, constipation, diarrhea, headache, dizziness, insomnia, palpitation, shortness of breath, mastitis, etc.

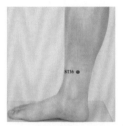

三阴交（SP6）
Sanyinjiao

2. 三阴交（SP6）Sanyinjiao

【定位】在小腿内侧，内踝尖上 3 寸，胫骨内侧缘后际。

【Location】On the inner side of the lower leg, 3 *cun* above the tip of the medial malleolus, on the posterior border of the medial margin of the tibia.

【主治】长期按摩三阴交穴可治疗腹胀、腹泻、肠鸣、月经不调、崩漏、水肿、小便不利、不孕、疝气、下肢痿痹等。

【Indications】Long-term massage of Sanyinjiao can treat abdominal distension, diarrhea, rumbling intestines, irregular menstruation, metrorrhagia, edema, adverse urination, infertility, hernia, lower limb paralysis and so on.

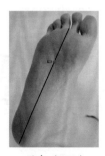

涌泉（KI1）
Yongquan

3. 涌泉（KI1）Yongquan

【定位】在足底，第 2、3 趾蹼缘与足跟连线的前 1/3 与后 2/3 的交点处。

【Location】On the sole of the foot, in a depression between the second and the third metatarsal bones, at the junction of the anterior one-third and the posterior two-thirds of the sole.

【主治】按摩该穴可防治失眠、健忘、高血压、中风、小便不利、咽喉肿痛等。

【Indications】Massaging this point can prevent and treat insomnia, forgetfulness, hypertension, stroke, adverse urination, sore throat, etc.

4. 太冲（LR3）Taichong

【定位】在足背，第1、2跖骨间，跖骨底结合部前方凹陷中，或触及动脉搏动。

【Location】On the dorsum of the foot, between the first and the second metatarsals, in the depression in front of the metatarsal base junction, or touch the arterial pulse.

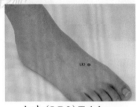

太冲（LR3）Taichong

【主治】常用于治疗脑血管病、高血压、面神经炎、青光眼、癫痫、肋间神经痛、月经不调等。

【Indications】It is commonly used to treat cerebrovascular disease, hypertension, facial neuritis, glaucoma, epilepsy, intercostal neuralgia, irregular menstruation and so on.

三、常见按摩手法介绍 Introduction to Common Massage Techniques

（一）揉法 Kneading method（ROU）

用手掌或手指在皮肤特定部位或穴位上做轻柔缓和的回旋揉动，带动该处的皮下组织，这就是揉法。揉法又可细分为掌揉法、指揉法。

Use the palms or fingers to make gentle rotary kneading on specific parts of the skin or acupoints to drive the subcutaneous tissue there, and this is called kneading method. Kneading

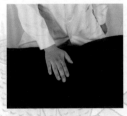

掌揉法
Palm kneading method

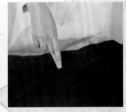

指揉法
Finger kneading method

method can be subdivided into palm kneading method and finger kneading method.

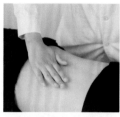

掌摩法 Palm rubbing method

（二）摩法 Rubbing method（MO）

用手掌或手指在体表做直线往返或环旋的摩擦运动，此法是按摩手法中最轻柔的一种，力道仅达皮肤及皮下组织。摩法又分为掌摩法和指摩法两种。

Use the palms or fingers to make a straight-line back and forth or circular friction movement on the body surface. This method is the gentlest of massage techniques, and its force only reaches the skin and the subcutaneous tissue. There are two types of rubbing methods: palm rubbing and finger rubbing.

（三）按法 Pressing method（AN）

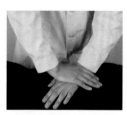

掌按法 Palm pressing method

用手指或手掌面着力在体表一定部位或穴位上，逐渐用力下压，这是最常见的按摩手法，动作简单。按法又可分为指按法、掌按法、肘按法。

Use the fingers or palms to focus on certain parts or acupoints on the body surface and gradually press down. This is the most common massage technique with simple action. Pressing method can be divided into finger pressing method, palm pressing method and elbow pressing method.

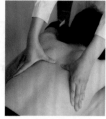

指推法 Finger pushing method

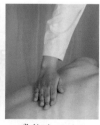

掌推法 Palm pushing method

（四）推法 Pushing method（TUI）

用手指或手掌着力于体表一定部位或穴位上，做单方向的直线或弧线移动。推法又可分为指推法、掌推法和肘推法。

Use the fingers or palms on certain parts or acupoints on the body surface to move in a straight line or arc in one direction. Pushing method can be divided into finger pushing method, palm pushing method and elbow pushing method.

（五）捏法、拿法 Pinching method, grasping method（NIE, NA）

捏法是利用拇指和其他手指在受术部位做对称性挤压；拿法是用拇指和其余手指的指端相对用力，拿住皮肤或肌肉，向上提起，随后再放下。

The pinching method is to use the thumb and other fingers to make symmetrical extrusion at the operation site. The grasping method is to use the thumb and the fingertips of other fingers to hold the skin or muscle, lift it up, and then put it down, exerting relative force.

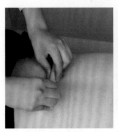 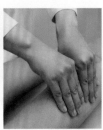

捏法 Pinching method   拿法 Grasping method

四、常见病的自我保健按摩 Self-care Massage for Common Diseases

（一）眼部保健 Eye care

1. 按揉穴位 Press and knead acupoints

两手握拳，用食指指腹在眼周按揉睛明、四白、丝竹空等穴，力度轻重适宜，每穴约 30 秒。反复操作 3~5 次，至眼部有热胀感即可。

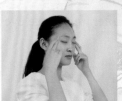

按揉穴位 Press and knead acupoints

Clench the fists with both hands, press and knead Jingming, Sibai, Sizhukong and other acupoints around the eyes with the index fingers for about 30 seconds with the appropriate intensity. Repeat the operation for 3–5 times until the eyes feel warm and swollen.

2. 按摩眼周 Press and rub around the eyes

两手掌心相对，大拇指按于两侧太阳穴，反过来用两手食指从内眼角

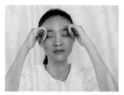

按摩眼周
Press and rub around
the eyes

处开始，沿着眼眶向两侧轻轻刮摩至太阳穴 20~30 次。

With the palms of both hands facing each other, the thumbs are pressed on the temples on both sides, and in turn, the index fingers of both hands are used to gently scrape and rub from the inner corner of the eye to both sides along the orbit to the temples for 20–30 times.

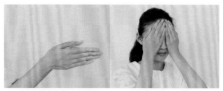

摩掌熨目 Rub the hands and iron the eyes

3. 摩掌熨目 Rub the hands and iron the eyes

手掌互相摩擦，搓热之后，将双手掌心放置于双眼之上，令眼部有温热舒适感。如此反复三次。如果能够在熨目之后再用手指轻轻按压眼球片刻，效果会更好。

Rub the palms against each other until you feel warm, and place the palms of both hands over the eyes to make them warm and comfortable. Repeat this operation three times. Press the eyeballs gently with the fingers for a moment after ironing the eyes for a better effect.

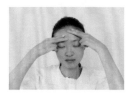

直推前额 Push straight
on the forehead

（二）头晕头痛 Dizziness and headache

1. 直推前额 Push straight on the forehead

用双手手指自两眉之间印堂至前发际做直推法 20~30 次，其余手指置于头的两侧相对固定。

Use the fingers of both hands to push straight from the Yintang between the eyebrows to the front hairline for 20–30 times, and the other fingers are placed on both sides of the head to fix relatively.

2. 按揉头面部穴位 Press and knead around scalp and facial acupoints

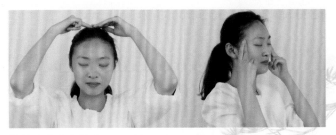

按揉头面部穴位 Press and knead around scalp and facial acupoints

用中指按揉百会穴，先按压 5 秒，再沿顺时针方向揉 25 秒，重复 3 次。随后以两手食指按在双太阳穴，先沿顺时针方向揉 30 秒，再逆时针揉 30 秒。

Press and knead Baihui with the middle finger. First press for 5 seconds, then knead clockwise for 25 seconds, and repeat three times. Then press the index fingers of both hands on the temples, knead clockwise for 30 seconds, and then counterclockwise for 30 seconds.

3. 按揉风池 Press and knead Fengchi

用双手的中指按在两侧风池穴，先按穴位 5 秒，再按顺时针方向揉穴位 10 秒，再从风池穴向下沿颈椎擦至颈肩。

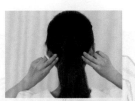

按揉风池 Press and knead Fengchi

Use the middle fingers of both hands to press on Fengchi on both sides for 5 seconds, then rub the acupoints clockwise for 10 seconds, and then rub the cervical vertebra down from Fengchi to the neck and shoulders.

（三）颈部不适 Neck discomfort

1. 按揉风池 Press and knead Fengchi

用双手拇指分别按在两侧风池穴，其余手指附在头的两侧，由轻到重地按揉 20~30 次。

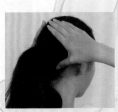

按揉风池 Press and knead Fengchi

Use the thumb of each hand to press on Fengchi on both sides, and attach the other fingers to both sides of the

127

head. Press and knead 20–30 times from light to heavy.

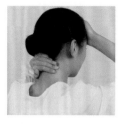

拿捏颈肌 Pinch and grasp the neck muscle

2. 拿捏颈肌 Pinch and grasp the neck muscle

用一只手扶住自己的前额，另一只手上举置于颈后，拇指放置于同侧颈外侧，其余四指放在颈肌对侧，双手用力对合，将颈肌向上提起后放松，沿风池穴向下拿捏至大椎穴 20~30 次。

Hold the forehead with one hand, raise the other hand to the back of the neck, place the thumb on the outside of the neck on the same side, put the other four fingers on the opposite side of the neck muscle, press the hands together, lift the neck muscles upwards and then relax them, and then grasp and pinch them down along Fengchi to Dazhui for 20–30 times.

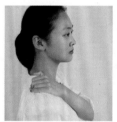

按揉肩颈 Press and knead shoulders and the neck

3. 按揉肩颈 Press and knead shoulders and the neck

按压颈部、背部肌肉约 2 分钟，最后拍打肩背及上肢部约 2 分钟。

Press the muscles of the neck and the back for about 2 minutes, and finally flap the shoulders, the back and the upper limbs for about 2 minutes.

（四）感冒 Cold

1. 按揉穴位 Press and knead acupoints

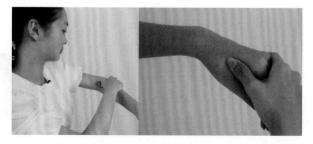

按揉穴位 Press and knead acupoints

按揉大椎、风池、尺泽、合谷等穴位，力度轻重适宜，每穴约 30 秒。反复操作 3~5 次。

Press and knead Dazhui, Fengchi, Chize, Hegu and other acupoints 30 seconds for each with appropriate strength. Repeat the operation for 3–5 times.

2. 按揉鼻部 Press and knead the nose

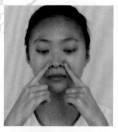

用手指尖按压迎香穴，一边按一边振动，直到达到酸胀感为止，每次 5~10 分钟。

Press Yingxiang with the tips of the fingers and vibrate them at the same time until it reaches the feeling of acid swelling, 5–10 minutes each time.

按揉鼻部 Press and knead the nose

3. 捻揉耳郭 Twirl and knead the auricle

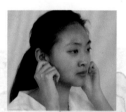

以拇指、食指对耳垂及耳郭进行捻揉，并向下拽摇耳垂，使耳道内部产生烘热感。

Twirl and knead the earlobe and the auricle with the thumb and the index finger, and drag and shake the earlobe downward to make the inner part of the ear canal hot.

捻揉耳郭 Twirl and knead the auricle

任务分析 Task Analysis

1. 请说出下列图片中穴位的中英文名称。

Please give the Chinese and English name of the acupoints in the following pictures.

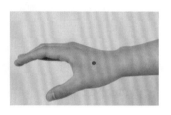 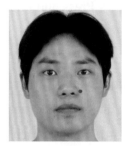

_____   _____

_____   _____

2. 请设计一套感冒自我保健按摩操。

Please design a set of self-care massage exercises for cold.

_____

_____

第四节 "神罐"之角法

Section 4 Magical Cupping—Cupping Therapy

学习情境描述 Learning Situation Description

根据实训室内提供的不同种类罐具，学习各种拔罐方法及其操作技术。

According to different kinds of cupping devices provided in the training room, learn various cupping methods and operation techniques.

学习目标 Learning Objectives

能够运用拔罐技术进行常见疾病的保健预防。

To be able to use the cupping technique for the health care and the prevention of common diseases.

任务导入 Task Import

拔罐法古称"角法"，是一种以罐为工具，利用燃烧、抽吸、蒸汽等方法造成罐内负压，使罐吸附于体表腧穴或患处一定部位，使皮肤充血、瘀血产生良性刺激，以达到防治疾病目的的一种中医外治法。

Cupping method, known as Horn method in ancient times, is a kind of external treatment method of Traditional Chinese Medicine, which takes the pot as a tool, uses combustion, suction, steam and other methods to create negative pressure in the pot, makes the pot adsorb on the acupoints on the body surface or a certain part of the affected part, and causes skin congestion and blood stasis to produce benign stimulation, so as to achieve the purpose of preventing and treating diseases.

一、罐具的种类与特点 Types and Characteristics of Cups

罐具的种类很多，目前临床常用的有玻璃罐、竹罐和抽气罐。

There are many kinds of cups. At present, glass jars, bamboo cups and suction cups are commonly used in clinic.

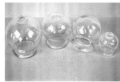

玻璃罐 Glass jar

（一）玻璃罐 Glass jar

由耐热、质硬的透明玻璃加工制成，形如球，罐口平滑。

It is made of heat-resistant and hard transparent glass, shaped like a ball, with a smooth jar mouth.

优点：质地透明，可观察罐内皮肤瘀血程度，以便掌握治疗时间。

Advantages: The transparent texture allows doctors to observe the level of skin stasis in the jar so as to control the duration of treatment.

缺点：易摔碎、易烫伤。

Disadvantages: Easy to break and scald.

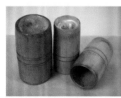

竹罐 Bamboo cup

（二）竹罐 Bamboo cup

用直径 3~5 厘米的竹子，制成 6~10 厘米长的竹筒，打磨至罐口光滑平整。

Using bamboos with a diameter of 3–5 cm to make a bamboo tube with a length of 6–10 cm, and polish it until the mouth of the pot is smooth and flat.

优点：取材容易，制作简单，轻巧价廉，不易摔碎。

Advantages: Easy to get the materials, simple to make, light and cheap, not easy to break.

缺点：容易爆裂漏气，吸拔力不大，质地不透明，难以观察罐内皮肤变化。

Disadvantages: It is easy to burst and leak, with small suction and extraction force. It is difficult to observe the changes of skin in the container because of its opaque texture.

（三）抽气罐 Suction cup

用透明塑料制成，其规格大小不同，顶部加置活塞，配合抽气筒使用。

It is made of transparent plastic with different specifications and sizes. A piston is added on it to cooperate with the air pump.

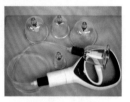

抽气罐 Suction cup

优点：可控制吸力，使用方便，操作简单，不易烫伤。

Advantages: Suction can be controlled, easy to use, simple to operate, and avoid scalding.

缺点：缺乏温热刺激，容易老化变形。

Disadvantages: Lack of warm stimulation, easy to aging and deformation.

无论选择哪一种罐具，罐口一定要圆滑、宽厚，以免在使用时伤及皮肤。

No matter which kind of cupping device is selected, pay attention to that the mouth must be smooth and wide so as not to hurt the skin in the course of cupping.

二、拔罐法的作用 Functions of Cupping

拔罐法具有祛风除湿、温经散寒、活血化瘀、消肿止痛、温阳益气等作用。

Cupping has the functions of dispelling wind and eliminating dampness, warming meridians and dispersing cold, quickening the blood and transforming stasis, dispersing swelling and relieving pain, warming *yang* and boosting *qi*.

现代研究表明，拔罐法的机械刺激和温热作用可有效促进血液循环和新陈代谢，从而调节神经系统功能，调节肌肉及关节活动，缓解机体疼痛，改善功能状态，从而达到防治疾病和强身健体的作用。

Modern research has shown that the mechanical stimulation and warming effect of cupping can effectively promote blood circulation and metabolism, so as to regulate the function of nervous system, regulate muscle and joint activities, relieve body pain, improve functional state, and then prevent and treat diseases and strengthen the body.

三、拔罐法的适应证和禁忌证 Indications and Contraindications of Cupping

（一）适应证 Indications

拔罐法的适应范围非常广泛，一般多用于风寒湿痹、腰背腿痛、关节痛、软组织闪挫扭伤及伤风感冒、头痛、咳嗽、腹痛腹泻、痛经、中风偏瘫、面瘫、痤疮、荨麻疹、肥胖等。目前，拔罐法已成为一种常用的保健疗法。

Cupping method has a wide range of adaptability. It is generally used for wind cold dampness arthralgia, low back and leg pain, joint pain, soft tissue flash, contusion and sprain, cold, headache, cough, abdominal pain, diarrhea, dysmenorrhea, stroke hemiplegia, facial paralysis, acne, urticaria, obesity, etc. It has become a common health care therapy.

（二）禁忌证 Contraindications

因全身发热而引起的头痛、抽搐、痉挛者。

Headache, convulsion and spasm caused by systemic fever.

各种皮肤病、溃疡、水肿者。

Various skin diseases, ulcers and edema.

孕妇的腰骶部和腹部以及大血管分布部位。

The lumbosacral and abdomen of pregnant women and the part with the distribution of large blood vessels.

四、拔罐方法 Cupping Method

（一）施术前准备 Preparation before cupping

患者准备：患者信息、操作适宜、皮肤、体位。

Patients preparation: Patients' information, appropriate operation, skin and body position.

物品准备：治疗盘、打火机、95% 酒精棉球、镊子或止血钳、凡士林、棉签、纱布等。

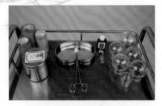

Materials preparation: Treatment plates, lighters, 95% alcohol cotton balls, forceps or hemostatic forceps, vaseline, cotton swabs, gauzes, etc.

物品准备 Materials preparation

环境准备：温度适宜、隐私保护。

Environmental preparation: Appropriate temperature and privacy protection.

医生准备：仪表整齐，洗手、戴口罩。

Doctors preparation: Tidy appearance. Wash hands and wear a mask.

（二）拔罐操作流程 Cupping processes

1. 拔罐 Cupping

一手持火罐，另一手持镊子或止血钳夹住 95% 的酒精棉球点燃，伸入罐内中下端绕 1 周或 2 周后迅速抽出。

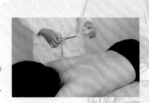

拔罐 Cupping

One hand holds the fire pot, the other hand holds forceps or hemostatic forceps to clamp 95% alcohol cotton ball for ignition, stretch into the middle and lower ends of the pot, and quickly pull it out after winding for 1 or 2 turns.

2. 留罐 Retaining cupping

迅速将罐口扣在选定部位上不动，确定吸牢后，留置 10~15 分钟。待施术部位皮肤充血或瘀血呈紫红色为度。

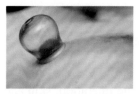

留罐 Retaining cupping

Quickly snap the jar mouth on the selected body part without moving it and leave it for 10–15 minutes after making sure that it is firmly sucked. Wait until the skin congestion or blood stasis at the operation site is purplish red.

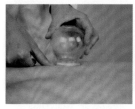

起罐 Removing cupping

3. 起罐 Removing cupping

最后左手夹住火罐向一侧稍微倾斜，右手拇指或食指、中指按压罐口皮肤，使空气进入罐内，即可将罐取下。

Finally, hold the cupping jar with the left hand and tilt it slightly to one side. Press the skin at the mouth of the jar with the right thumb or the index finger and the middle finger to make air enter the jar and remove it.

（三）整理调复 Arranging, adjusting and restoring

协助患者整理衣物、整理床单和物品等。嘱患者休息片刻，拔罐局部要避风寒，2 小时内不要洗浴。将用过的罐具、止血钳等进行消毒，以备下次治疗使用。

Assist the patient in tidying up their clothes; make up the sheets, articles, etc. Ask the patient to rest for a while, keep warm, avoid wind and cold in the cupping part, and not to take a bath within 2 hours. Disinfect the used containers and hemostatic forceps for the next treatment.

五、拔罐的注意事项 Cautions for Cupping

拔罐时，要选择适当体位和肌肉相对丰满的部位。若体位不当，或骨骼凹凸不平、毛发较多的部位，罐具易脱落。

Choose the appropriate body position and the part with relatively plump muscles. If the body position is improper, or the parts have uneven bones and thick hair, the cups are easy to fall off.

拔罐前要根据所拔部位的大小选择尺寸适宜的罐，使用前检查罐口是否平整、光滑，竹罐要检查是否有裂隙，以免漏气。

Before cupping, select cups with appropriate size according to the size of the body part. Check whether the cups' mouth is flat and smooth before use. Check whether there are cracks in the bamboo tank to avoid air leakage.

拔罐手法要熟练，动作要轻、快、稳、准，注意用火安全。

The cupping technique should be skilled, and the action should be light, fast, stable and accurate. Pay attention to the safety use of fire.

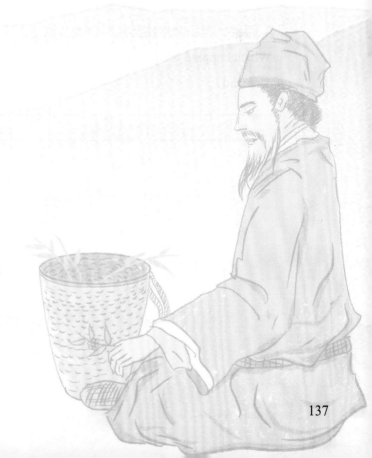

任务分析 Task Analysis

1.描述常用罐具的种类和特点以及临床使用时该如何选择。

Describe the types and characteristics of commonly used cups and how to choose them in clinical use.

_____

_____

2.常用罐的吸拔方法有哪些？临床该如何运用？

What are the suction and extraction methods of common cups? How should they be used clinically?

_____

_____

3.腰背、大腿部疼痛且范围较大，该选用哪种拔罐方式？

Which cupping method should be used for the low back and thigh pain that is widespread?

_____

_____

第五节 "中国功夫"之养生功法

Section 5 Chinese Kungfu—Traditional Chinese Exercise for Health Preservation

学习情境描述 Learning Situation Description

以教师示教、实践操作为主，理论讲解为辅，学习中华传统养生功法的相关知识。

Based on teacher's teaching demonstration and practical operation, supplemented by theoretical explanation, learn the relevant knowledge of traditional Chinese health preservation skills.

学习目标 Learning Objectives

了解养生与养生功法的概念，领会养生功法的内在特点。

To know the concepts of health preservation and health preservation exercise, and understand the internal characteristics of health preservation exercise.

任务导入 Task Import

一、中华传统养生功法 Chinese Traditional Health Preservation Exercise

中华传统养生功法，是指在祖国传统医学理论指导下，通过一定的技巧动作、呼吸吐纳、意念导引等，达到强身健体、增强免疫、延年益寿的特殊方法。旧称"导引""按跷"，是我国古代劳动人民在长期生活实践中创造并总结的自我身心锻炼的健身方法，有着悠久的历史和广泛的群众基础。其内容形式丰富，流传至今的有八段锦、易筋经、五禽戏、太极拳、六字诀等。

Chinese traditional health preservation exercise is a special exercise under the guidance of Traditional Chinese Medicine theory. This exercise uses some special actions, breathing methods, mind guidance and other methods to strengthen the body, enhance immunity and prolong life. Previously known as *daoyin* and *anqiao*, they are the fitness methods of self physical and mental exercise created and summarized by the working people in ancient China in their long-term life practice. It has a long history and a broad mass base. Its contents and forms are diverse, and the skill that have been completely spread to the present include Baduanjin, Yijinjing, Wuqinxi, Taijiquan, Liuzijue and so on.

练习养生功法的根本目的是强身健体、延年益寿，要达到这一目的，关键是遵循相应的练习原则，在合理选择功法的基础上，积极主动，形、气、神同调，循序渐进，持之以恒，规范动作，养练结合，动静相宜。

The fundamental purpose of practicing traditional health preservation exercise is to strengthen the body and prolong life. The key to achieve this goal is to follow the corresponding practice principles, to be active on the basis of a reasonable choice of exercises, to harmonize the body, *qi* and spirit, to progress step by step, to be persistent, to standardize the movements, to combine nurturing and practising, and to move and be still.

二、常见功法介绍 Introduction to Common Traditional Health Preservation Exercise

（一）八段锦 Baduanjin

八段锦是历史悠久、流传广泛的传统养生功法，在魏晋时期的《灵剑子引导子午记》中就有相关记载。练习时躯体四肢与气息、调心相结合，动作简单易行，效果显著，自隋唐以来，深受我国人民喜爱。八段锦动作轻柔和缓，松紧动静相兼，健身效果好，易学、省时。经常进行这项运动可以强健器官和肌肉，预防和治疗脊柱相关疾患，防治心脑血管疾病等。

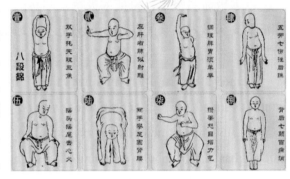

八段锦 Baduanjin

Baduanjin is a widely spread traditional health preservation exercise with a long history. It has been recorded in the *Lingjianzi Guiding Ziwuji* in the Wei-Jin Period. When practicing, people make the body and limbs combine with breath and mind adjustment. The movements are simple and easy to perform, and the effect is remarkable. It has been deeply loved by the Chinese people since the Sui and Tang Dynasties. Its movements are gentle and slow, elastic, dynamic and static. It is effective for keeping fit, easy to learn, and time-saving. Regular practice of this exercise can strengthen one's internal organs as well as one's muscles, prevent and treat spine related diseases, prevent cardiovascular and cerebrovascular diseases and so on.

（二）太极拳 Taijiquan

太极拳作为一项集健身与养生于一体的运动，其内涵博大精深、健身作用独特，在现代社会紧张、快节奏的氛围下更能体现其不可替代的作用。

太极拳 Taijiquan

Taijiquan, as a sport which integrates physical training and health-preserving, has rich connotation and unique fitness function, which can better show its irreplaceable role in the tense and fast-paced atmosphere of modern society.

以太极命名拳术，象征太极拳是圆转的、弧形的，是一阴一阳、刚柔相济的高深拳术，它的拳法、拳理包罗天地变化。其流派众多，流传比较广的主要有陈、杨、吴、武、孙等五大流派。

Named after Taiji, it symbolizes that Taijiquan is circular and curved. It is an advanced boxing technique of *yin and yang*, combining hardness and softness. Its boxing methods and principles include the changes of heaven and earth. It has many schools, including Chen, Yang, Wu, Wu and Sun.

长期练习太极拳既可强身健体，又可防治许多慢性疾病，是抗衰老最有效的措施。但有肺、肾、肝、胃急性炎症者应暂停练习。

Persisting in practicing Taijiquan can not only strengthen the body, but also prevent and treat many chronic diseases. It can slow down the rate of aging effectively. However, those with acute inflammation of the lung, the kidney, the liver and the stomach should stop practicing.

三、八段锦演练示范 Demonstration and Explanation of Baduanjin

（一）预备式 Ready position

两脚并步自然站立，身体中正，目视前方，松静自然，舌抵上腭，凝神调息，气沉丹田，鼻吸口呼。沉髋屈膝，重心微右移，左腿向左开步，与肩同宽，脚尖向前。两臂内旋外展，外旋前屈，两手虎口相对，在小腹前抱球，两掌之间间隔约10厘米。

Move the left foot from the right foot, stand restfully. Swing the arms forward in a circle, as if holding a hollow ball in front of the navel. Draw in the chin, the belly, and the buttocks to keep the torso straight. Bend the knees slightly and squat, breath naturally through the nose, with mind concentration on Dantian, which locates on the lower abdomen, on the anterior midline, a distance of four fingers below the umbilicus. Look ahead and close the mouth and teeth lightly with the tongue resting on the palate.

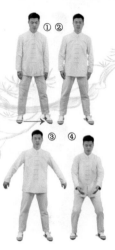

预备式
Ready position

（二）第一式 双手托天理三焦 Form 1 Holding up the hands high with palms up to regular *sanjiao*

预备式。（呼气）双手于小腹前交叉，缓缓上举，双手上举时两腿徐徐立直。双手到胸前内旋翻掌，掌心向上，（吸气）用力向上托举于头顶，同时抬头，目视两掌。（呼气）下颌内收，目视前方，十指分开，两臂分别从身体两侧下落于小腹前，掌心向上，同时身体重心缓缓下降，双膝微屈，回到预备式，稍停片刻，调整呼吸。以上为1遍，如此反复6遍。

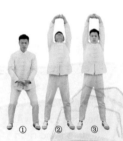

双手托天理三焦
Holding up the hands high with palms up to regular *sanjiao*

Follow the preparation form. Raise the hands overhead in front of the body with palms facing upward. Turn the palms when they pass by the face. Raise the hands up to the sky. Look upward while propping up. Return to the starting pose by lowering the arms sideways. Inhale while lifting hands and exhale while lowering them. This is one circle. Repeat 6 times.

（三）第二式 左右开弓似射雕 Form 2 Posing as an archer shooting eagle with both left and right hands

预备式。左足向左开大步，身体下蹲作马步。（吸气）

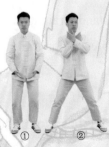

143

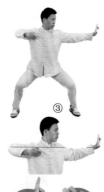

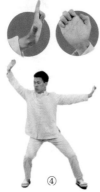

左右开弓似射雕
Posing as an archer
shooting eagle with
both left and right
hands

两臂上托在胸前交叉，掌心向内，左臂在外，右臂在内，右手各手指指间关节屈曲呈横掌，左手手掌直立做"箭指"（中指、无名指、小指指间关节屈曲，拇指、食指伸直，虎口撑开，呈八字掌）。（呼气）右肩后收，右手向右拉至右肩前，左手呈箭指向左推出，两手对抻作拉弓状。同时头随左手左转，目视左手食指，稍作停顿。

Follow the preparation form. Take a big step to the left. Adopt the horse stance. Lift hands, palms inward, and forearms crossed. Place the left hand on the wrist of the other. Bend the knees as if riding on a horse and drawing a bow. Stretch out the left arm with the index and the middle fingers erect and other fingers bent. Bend the right arm while making a fist and draw the elbow to the right side, as if drawing the bow. Hold on for a moment.

（吸气）重心上提，目视右掌，右手五指舒展，掌心向前，右臂向上向右画弧至与肩同高时，两手舒展，同时下落，至小腹前呈抱球状，目视前方。同时左足收回至与肩同宽，呈预备式。本式一左一右为1遍，共做3遍。

Repeat this movement to the other side. Inhale when drawing the bow and exhale when returning to the starting pose. Remember to keep the weight centered on the middle and withdraw the buttocks while drawing the bow. Repeat 3 times on both sides，hands apart. Withdraw the left foot to stand straight, with the feet apart at the end of the movement. Return to the preparation form.

（四）第三式 调理脾胃须单举 Form 3 Holding one arm overhead to modulate the function of the spleen and the stomach

预备式。（吸气）重心上提，双膝徐徐伸直，左手上举，掌心向上，至胸前旋腕（呼气），掌心向上，上托至头上方，肘关节微屈，四指并拢，指尖向右，用力上托，力达掌根；同时右手翻掌从身体前方下按至体侧，掌心向下，指尖向前。两手一上一下，互相争力。

Follow the preparation form. Lift the body up and straighten the knees slowly. Raise the left hand and put the four fingers together. When reaching the chest, rotate the wrist to keep the palm upward until it reaches above the

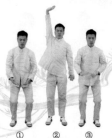

调理脾胃须单举
Holding one arm overhead to modulate the function of the spleen and the stomach

head. The palm root of the left hand is forced upward to hold the fingertip to the right, and the elbow joint is slightly flexed; at the same time, turn the palm of the right hand down from the front of the body to the side of the body, with the palm down and the fingertips forward. Push up one hand and press down the other to antagonize each other.

（吸气）松腰沉髋，重心缓缓下落至两膝关节微屈;同时左臂外旋翻掌，掌心向内，经身体前方缓缓下落至小腹前；右臂外旋上托，掌心向上，双手至腹部水平时重心上提，双膝徐徐伸直。（呼气）右手胸前旋腕上托至头上方，如此两侧交替反复进行。本式一左一右为1遍，共做3遍。第三遍结束时回到预备式。

Return to the starting posture by lowering the left hand in front of the body. Reverse the action by lifting the right hand. Inhale while lifting the arm and exhale while lowering the arm. Repeat 3 times on both sides, and return to the preparation form at the end of the movement.

（五）第四式 五劳七伤向后瞧 Form 4 Looking backward to prevent diseases due to the dysfunction of five *zang*-organs and seven-emotion disorders

预备式。双膝徐徐伸直，两手翻掌下按，指尖相对，于两髋前侧下按，

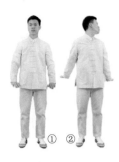

五劳七伤 向后瞧
Looking backward to prevent diseases due to the dysfunction of five *zang*-organs and seven-emotion disorders

肘关节微屈。（呼气）头缓缓向左后方观望，同时两手臂旋外，双手立腕下按，指尖朝向后方，稍停片刻。

Follow the preparation form. Lift the body up and straighten the knees slowly. Rotate the arms inward so that the palms are pressed down on the outside of the hips, the fingertips are forward, and the elbows are slightly flexed. Exhale and turn the head slowly to the left rear to look back and down. At the same time, rotate the shoulder joints back so that the fingertips point back. Press the hands down and extend the wrist back. Hold on for a moment.

（吸气）松腰沉髋，重心缓缓下移，两膝微屈；腕关节放松，手臂旋内，掌心向前回收，手臂旋前按掌于两髋前侧。如此两侧交替反复进行。本式一左一右为1遍，共做3遍。第三遍结束时回到预备式。

Inhale and turn the head to the front, relax and flex the hip joint, and slightly bend the knees to move the center of gravity down slowly. Turn the arms forward and press the palms on the outside of hips. Repeat 3 times on both sides, and return to the preparation form at the end of the movement.

（六）第五式 摇头摆尾去心火 Form 5 Swinging the head and lower the back to relieve the heart fire

预备式。左足向左横开大步，屈膝半蹲成马步。两手按在膝上部，虎口向内。（呼气）以腰为轴，将躯干转向左前方，屈髋带动上身向左前方俯身，目视左脚背，臀部向右后方作撑劲。（吸气）以腰

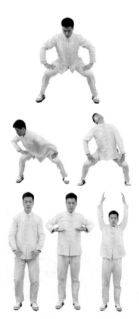

摇头摆尾去心火 Swinging the head and lower the back to relieve the heart fire

为轴，身体由左侧倾慢慢移动到右侧，目视右侧脚背。以髋为轴，上身缓缓抬起，随之抬头。左臂绷紧，右臂弯曲，以助摇摆。

Follow the preparation form. Take a big step to the left. Adopt the horse stance. Put the hands on the front of thighs with the fingertips facing each other. Exhale with the waist as the axis, and rotate the upper body to face the left front, so that the hip joint flexes. Tilt the upper body to the left front, look at the back of the left foot, and make the hips pout to the right rear. Inhale and take the waist as the axis. Slowly move the upper body from the left side to the right side, and look at the instep of the right side. With the hips as the axis, raises the upper body slowly and then looks up. Shake the body by tightening the left arm and bending the right arm.

（呼气）仰头向左侧转动头部，同时臀部向右侧摆动，至右侧弓步，上身面向左前方，目视左脚背，稍停片刻。上身转向右前方，屈髋带动上身向右前方俯身，动作同上，方向相反。两边交替反复进行。本式一左一右为1遍，共做3遍。第三遍结束时回到预备式。

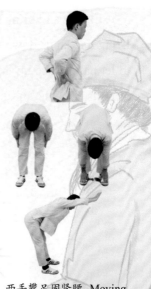

Exhale and raise the head and rotate the cervical spine to the left, while the hips swing to the right, with the legs stretching to the right. Turn the upper body to the front left, look at the back of the left foot and hold on for a moment. Repeat 3 times on both sides, and return to the preparation form at the end of the movement.

（七）第六式 两手攀足固肾腰 Form 6 Moving the hands from the armpit down to the feet to strengthen the kidney to prevent the lumber disorders

两手攀足固肾腰 Moving the hands from the armpit down to the feet to strengthen the kidney to prevent the lumber disorders

147

预备式。双下肢挺膝伸直，两手虎口相对，按于脐周，（吸气）双手向后摩运至肾俞穴。两手顺势沿脊柱两侧下摩至臀后，随之上体前倾，（呼气）双手继续沿膀胱经下摩至足跟，再向前攀足尖，意守涌泉穴，稍停片刻。（吸气）两手向前伸展，带动上身起立，缓缓直腰，双手上举，掌心向前，目视前方。

Follow the preparation form. Straighten the legs slowly and put the hands opposite to each other around the navel. Inhale and move the hands outward to the back. Rub the hands along the sides of the spine to the hips, and then lean forward. Exhale and then move the hands further down along the back of the thigh to the arch of the feet. Lift the hands laterally while inhaling.

（呼气）两臂旋外至掌心相对，缓缓下落，于胸前翻掌，从腋下向后摩运至背部脊柱两侧。（吸气）两手顺势沿脊柱两侧下摩至臀后，其后动作同上，反复6遍。结束时回到预备式。

Exhale and bring the hands down. Lift the hands forward. Bend the elbows. Bring the hands down to the front of the chest. Inhale and turn the arms outward to let palms face up. Move the hands to the back of the upper body through the armpits. Exhale and move the hands along the sides of the spine to the hips, further down along the back of the thigh to the arch of the feet. The routine should be done 6 times, and return to the preparation form at the end of the movement.

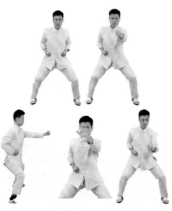

攒拳怒目增气力 Thrusting the fists and making the eyes glare to enhance strength

（八）第七式　攒拳怒目增气力
Form 7　Thrusting the fists and making the eyes glare to enhance strength

预备式。（吸气）左足平开屈膝成马步，两手握拳，立拳放于腰侧，拳眼向上，拳心向内，意守丹田。（呼气）左拳用力向前方缓缓击出，同时双目虎视出拳方向。左臂伸直，拳心向下，由拳变掌，（吸气）收回左拳，如法击出右拳，左右交替进行，各做 3 遍。结束时两拳松开，（吸气）双臂由体侧向上画弧至上方（呼气）缓缓下落，同时收回左足，回到预备式。

Follow the preparation form. Take a big step sideway to the left. Adopt the horse stance. Drop the torso with fists beside the waist. Thrust the clenched left fist slowly forward using internal force. Turn the hand and then grab and withdraw the punched- out fist. Punch the two fists in turn. Inhale when withdrawing the fist and exhale when punching. Clench the teeth tightly and open the eyes wide with the state of anger. Toes should grip the ground firmly. Do not protrude the buttocks and pull in the lower back. Repeat 3 times on both sides，and return to the preparation form at the end of the movement.

（九）第八式 背后七颠百病消 Form 8 Raising and lowering the heels seven times to prevent diseases

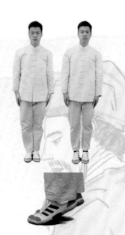

背后七颠百病消
Raising and lowering the heels seven times to prevent diseases

预备式。两腿并拢，立正放松，目视前方。（吸气）重心略前移，两足跟提起，前脚掌支撑身体，咬牙，舌抵上腭，头上顶，稍作停顿。（呼气）足跟缓缓下落，身体放松，保持舌抵上腭，足跟下落着地，轻震地面，如此反复 7 次。

Follow the preparation form. Stand straight with the legs together and the hands on the sides. Stand at ease and look ahead. Lift the heels and raise the body. Lower down the heels to tap them on the ground to give the body a little shock. Inhale while lifting the heels and exhale while lowering them. For those who are not very strong, lower the heels gently. The head should be kept erect to prevent too much shock to the cervical vertebrae. This is the last form of the routine. The routine should be done 7 times.

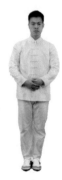

（十）收势　Form end

上式结束时，双臂外展至两手与髋同高，两臂屈肘，叠掌置于丹田处（男性左手在内，女性右手在内），目视前方，意守丹田，平静呼吸。调整呼吸后，两手自然下落。收势后可行搓手浴面，肢体放松等整理动作，不可急于走动。

收势 Form end

After the last routine, turn the palms outwards, overlap the palms in front of Dantian and look ahead. Adjust the breathing rhythm and relax for a while before finishing. Then hands down, finished. After finishing, rub hands to cover the face and do limb relaxation. Do not rush to vigorous activities.

任务分析 Task Analysis

1. 说出八段锦的功法特点及练习要领。

Please tell the characteristics of Baduanjin and the key points when practicing it.

_____

_____

2. 跟随口令音乐及实操演示，练习八段锦。

Please follow the instructions, music and practical demonstration to practice Baduanjin.

_____

_____

3. 说出八段锦的每一段的动作特点及各自的养生作用。

Please explain the movement characteristics of each section of Baduanjin and their health preservation functions.

_____

_____